PARKINSON'S DISEASE RECLAIM YOUR LIFE

Tips To Help Manage Your Symptoms

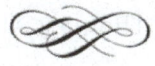

Susha Thomas PT, DPT, C/NDT

Disclaimer: The material provided in this book is for educational and informational purposes only. Always seek the advice of your physician and/or other qualified health care providers with any questions you may have regarding treatment that is best for you. The names and cases used in this book do not represent actual people or events. Any resemblances to actual events or persons are entirely coincidental.

©2022 Susha Thomas. All rights reserved.

Dedication

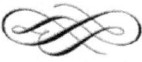

This book is dedicated to my mom, Saramma Zacharia, whose unconditional love and support is always with me. She passed away from cancer at the young age of fifty-three, but in her short life on earth, she inspired many; she had a selfless spirit and being a nurse, served others throughout her life. Her laugh and presence would light up any room and she taught us the importance of a good work ethic and perseverance. She was thoughtful, kind, and had the most caring heart. Through the cancer, she fought valiantly and courageously, but humbly and quietly. She managed to find the good in all things. Her selfless love and dedication to others inspired me to write this book to inspire others to live their life to the fullest no matter what life throws at them.

TABLE OF CONTENTS

Introduction 1

Chapter 1: Parkinson's Explained 3

Chapter 2: I Think I May Have Parkinson's. What Do I Do? 9

Chapter 3: Common Medications for Parkinson's Explained 15

Chapter 4: My Brain Is Giving My Body the Wrong Messages and Making My World Smaller 19

Chapter 5: I Am Losing My Voice 24

Chapter 6: My Handwriting is Getting Smaller 30

Chapter 7: It's So Hard to Roll and Move Around in Bed 34

Chapter 8: I'm Stuck, and I Can't Stand Up 37

Chapter 9: My Steps are Smaller, and I Shuffle Them When I Walk 41

Chapter 10: Dressing Myself and Combing My Hair is Taking Longer Than It Should 48

Chapter 11: When I Get Up, I Get Dizzy, and My Blood Pressure Suddenly Drops 55

Chapter 12: My Tremors Make It Hard for Me to Eat with a Spoon 60

Chapter 13: I Fall More Often Now 65

Chapter 14: What Home Modifications Do I Need? 71

Chapter 15: My Memory is Getting Worse 79

Chapter 16: I Am Stooping, and My Posture is Getting Worse 84

Chapter 17: I Have a Referral for Physical Therapy, Occupational Therapy and Speech Therapy 86

Chapter 18: My Therapist Recommended I Join a Gym and Do Aerobic Exercise 93

Chapter 19: Reclaim Your Life and Don't Give Up 96

Chapter 20: You've Got This! 98

Resources 101

References 109

About the Author: 116

Index 117

Introduction

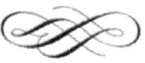

Approximately 60,000 Americans are diagnosed with Parkinson's Disease every year, and more than 10 million people are affected worldwide. Even though Parkinson's is a progressive disorder, there is so much you can do to help slow and manage your symptoms. This book provides insight from the perspective of a Physical Therapist on Parkinson's disease and expands on why the symptoms appear and what can be done to help manage them. From freezing with walking to small handwriting to a soft voice, there is so much you can do to help manage symptoms! The only proven thing that can slow the progression of the disease is exercise, and this book provides suggestions on exercises that are beneficial with Parkinson's. It provides strategies and tips for patients and caregivers to improve daily function and quality of life and provides in-depth recommendations on adaptive equipment and home modifications that can be used to improve independence with daily tasks. It details not only how to reduce symptoms but also goes into the neurological mechanisms behind the symptoms. By stepping out of your comfort zone and incorporating exercise and the other helpful tips in this book, you will make steady progress and notice the difference in your daily activities. In my experience treating Parkinson's patients, several of them had given up hope and were in despair because they felt like there was not anything they could do to help manage their symptoms. But when they started using the tips, tricks, and strategies that I provided them, they were amazed at how much they could do! This inspired me to jot down my suggestions and compose it into a book because I realized there are still more out there that have lost all hope. With this book, I hope to make a positive impact in the life of at least one person who has been affected by Parkinson's. Whether you are newly diagnosed or have had Parkinson's for several years, this book will give you the tips and tricks you need to regain independence in your daily life. Reclaim your life, you've got this!

Chapter 1:
Parkinson's Explained

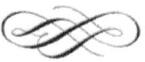

Sara is a healthy fifty-three-year-old woman who has big plans for her future. She loves spending time with her family, especially her grandchildren. She is fiercely independent. We will be talking more about Sara and her journey after being diagnosed with Parkinson's in this book.

Parkinson's is a progressive disease of the Central Nervous system that affects movement. More than 1.5 million people in the United States alone have Parkinson's. Some famous people you know have Parkinson's Disease including Michael J. Fox, Muhammad Ali, Ozzy Osbourne, Neil Diamond, and Billy Graham to name a few. So why does it occur? Deep in the brain there are parts called the substantia nigra and the basal ganglia. Why are these parts of the brain important to know about with Parkinson's? Well, the nerve cells in the substantia nigra produce a chemical (neurotransmitter) called dopamine. In Parkinson's, the level of dopamine is substantially reduced. So why is dopamine so important? As you may know, people living with Parkinson's have slowness of movement—their entire world suddenly becomes smaller. This is because dopamine is responsible for efficient movement. So, a decrease in dopamine means a decrease in the quality of movement, making everything smaller!

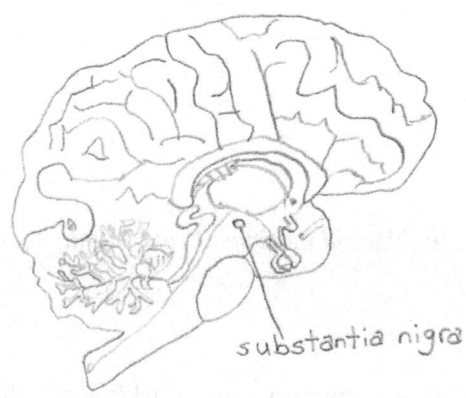

Figure 1a- Brain

Imagine a person who does not have Parkinson's reaching out for a phone that is on the couch. The level of dopamine in their brain is normal, and so their brain gives their muscles the correct message (or signal) to reach out exactly this far (say twelve inches), then open their hand and grab the phone.

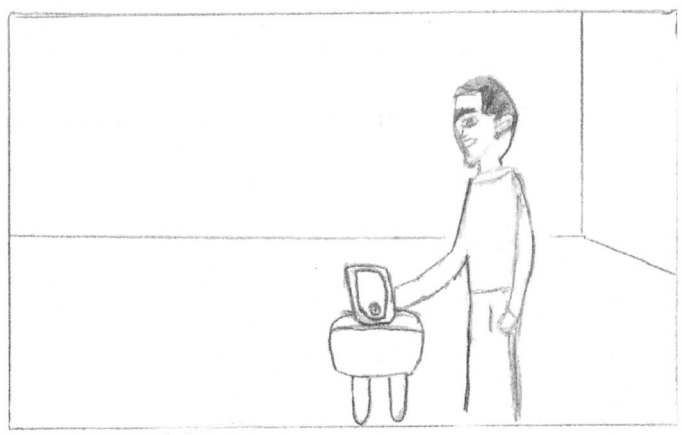

Figure 1b- Normal movement- picking up a phone

Now let's imagine a person with Parkinson's doing this same activity. The level of dopamine in the brain of a person with Parkinson's is less, so their brain gives their muscles a very weak message (or signal). So instead of reaching the needed twelve inches, maybe at around eight inches, the brain gives the muscles the wrong message, "Ok you have reached the object, you can stop reaching." But the movement stopped four inches shy of twelve inches, making it a much smaller movement. Therefore, everything seems smaller with Parkinson's—it's not their fault—the brain is giving the muscles the wrong message because of the decreased dopamine in their brain.

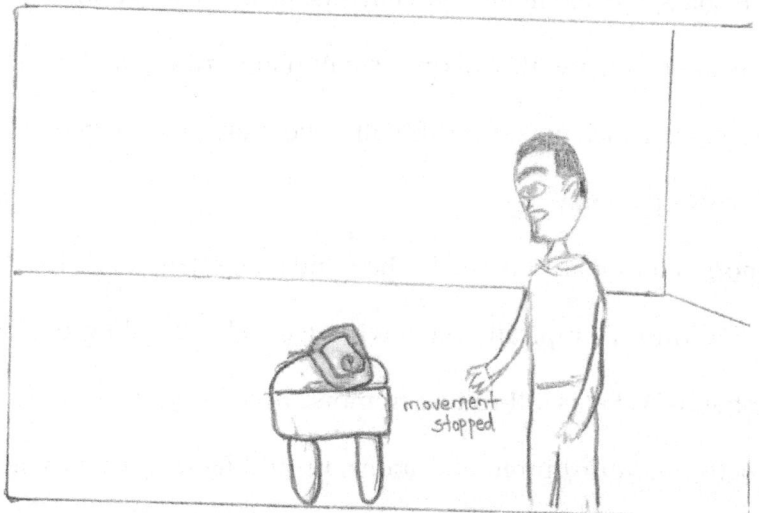

Figure 1c- Parkinson movement- smaller, undershooting target

Symptoms of Parkinson's begin to appear when around eighty percent of the chemical dopamine has been depleted. Imagine that eighty percent! That means that several people may have the beginning stages of Parkinson's but do not even know it for a good six years before their symptoms start to appear!

The classical symptoms of Parkinson's are smaller movements, tremors, rigidity, and poor balance. Let's dig into each of these symptoms and try to understand them more.

Smaller movements: Why the smaller movements? Yes, it is because normal dopamine means normal movements, lesser dopamine (as in Parkinson's) means smaller movements. People with Parkinson's will notice small steps with walking, small handwriting, and smaller or lower voice which makes it difficult to be understood when carrying out a conversation.

Tremors: Tremors can occur in the hands, legs, jaw, or head. People with Parkinson's typically have what we call pill-rolling tremors in their hands. What is pill-rolling tremors? Imagine you had a medicine pill between your thumb and index, or middle finger and you kept rolling that pill between your fingers. That is what pill-rolling tremors look like. These are involuntary movements which means that the person does not intentionally have tremors, it just comes and goes.

Rigidity: What is rigidity? In simple words it means stiffness. The muscles start to get stiff resulting in poor posture, rounded shoulders, bent back and difficulty moving around.

Poor balance: Poor balance and impaired coordination are key features of the disease that could lead to falls.

Parkinson's is a progressive disorder, but there are things you can do to help manage the symptoms and slow the progression of the disease. The following chapters will highlight tips and exercises that can be incorporated into your daily routine to improve your independence with daily activities and help manage your symptoms.

Chapter 2
I Think I May Have Parkinson's. What Do I Do?

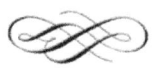

Sara woke up one morning and something did not feel right. She just woke up; the room was still dark, and her alarm hadn't gone off yet. She wondered to herself, 'Why am I feeling stiff? I feel like I can't move.' With extra time, Sara got out of bed. She went over to the office where she needed to write some checks to pay some pending bills. She glanced at the checks written and notices how bad her handwriting has gotten; she could barely read what she wrote as it was so small and cramped. Sara thought back and realized that within the past several months, things were getting harder, and it was taking longer for her to do everyday tasks. She thought to herself, 'Is it time to go see a doctor and find out what's going on?'

Early symptoms of the disease are very subtle and if you don't pay attention, you may just brush it off.

People with Parkinson's ask themselves some of the below questions:

- Is my voice getting softer? Why can't my family hear what I am saying?
- Is my handwriting getting smaller? Why can't I write out a check anymore? Why is my handwriting so difficult to read?
- I feel stuck to the floor when I try to walk or turn, how come?
- Why is it getting harder to get out of bed?
- Why is it taking longer to do my normal activities like brushing my teeth and combing my hair?
- Why is my hand shaking?
- I have been told that my face looks serious, depressed, and emotionless—a masked face, why?
- I feel like I'm off balance, what's happening?
- Buttoning my shirt is getting harder and harder, why?
- My sense of smell isn't that great anymore, what's going on?
- I am having a hard time remembering things, is this normal?
- Why am I having a tough time sleeping?

- I am not standing up as straight as I used to and I am hunched over, is this old age?
- I started having constipation and my bowels are not moving regularly, why?
- I am having difficulty swallowing and I have started drooling at times, am I okay?

Consult your doctor if you are experiencing any of these signs; some of the signs may be the normal aging process or they could be signs of a problem like Parkinson's disease.

Your doctor may refer you to a neurologist—a doctor who specializes in and treats diseases of the brain and spinal cord. During your first appointment, your neurologist will perform a physical exam and a neurological exam. Your neurologist will test your muscle strength, reflexes, and sensation and ask you about any symptoms you may have been experiencing. Many neurologists also observe patients get out of a chair and have them walk to see if there are coordination problems, shuffling or small steps.

Detecting and diagnosing Parkinson's disease in its early stages can allow for greater treatment success and management of symptoms. Unfortunately, there is still no cure for Parkinson's, but the earlier it is detected, the sooner treatment can start and help improve quality of life. Remember how we talked about that chemical in the brain called dopamine that controls movement and how there is less of it present in Parkinson's? Well, if your neurologist suspects you have Parkinson's, they may start you on medications that substitute the lost dopamine (example: Medications like Carbidopa/Levodopa®-DOPA is short for dopamine, dopamine agonists, amantadine®, etc.) and see if these medications are helping with the symptoms. If they are, then your doctor may diagnose you with Parkinson's. As these levels now increase, brain function will become better, and a patient may experience fewer symptoms associated with Parkinson's. Regular checkups with your neurologist are required because your body may develop a tolerance to the medications and in that case, adjustments to dosage or changing medications may be warranted.

If traditional medications are not working, your neurologist may prescribe a surgical procedure called Deep Brain Stimulation. This is an implantable neurostimulation system that targets a specific area of the brain called the Substantia Nigra. The DBS has shown to be effective in managing symptoms like stiffness, slowness, shuffling gait or freezing. It may also help to control involuntary muscle contractions that cause repetitive or twisting movements (dystonia) and involuntary movements (dyskinesia).

Duopa® enteral suspension is a prescription medicine used for the treatment of advanced Parkinson's disease. Your neurologist will recommend this treatment approach if it is right for you. Duopa® contains two medicines: carbidopa® and levodopa®. Duopa® is delivered right into the intestine, so your levodopa can be absorbed quickly. This approach does require surgery as the medication port needs to be placed in the stomach. Your doctor will then place a portable pump for the continuous delivery of levodopa, lessening the need for oral pills.

Your doctor may also talk to you about your diet and encourage you to keep hydrated and drink more water. Dehydration can cause low blood pressure which can result in you becoming faint and increases your risk of falling. It is important to drink at least eight eight-ounce glasses of water a day to help prevent constipation. They may also recommend eating foods rich in vitamin D and decreasing protein-rich foods as they may interfere with the medication's effectiveness.

If you have been newly diagnosed with Parkinson's your emotions may be all over the spectrum—don't worry, you're not alone. For some, the diagnosis may come as a relief as they have an answer for their previously unexplained symptoms. However, others may have a harder time processing this diagnosis and struggling with how they manage this information. There are a lot of things that you can do to maintain and improve your quality of life, so don't lose hope! The following chapters are designed to provide you with more insight into how to recognize and manage your symptoms.

Chapter 3
Common Medications for Parkinson's Explained

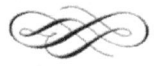

Sara pulled up to the neurologist's office. She sat in her car for several minutes, the keys still in the ignition. 'Was this the right decision? What if he gives me a diagnosis that I'm not ready for?' she thought to herself. She mustered up the courage and turned off the ignition, she took a deep breath and started walking into the doctor's office. The neurologist examined Sara. "I'd like to start you on a few Parkinson's medications to see if they will help with some of the symptoms you are describing. It's important that you take these medications on time every day." Sara's heart felt heavy, this was all so new to her. She could not process a lot of what the doctor explained after that, and her mind went blank. "Sara, do you understand the information I have given you? Do you have any questions," the doctor asked. Sara shook her head no as she slowly got up to leave her appointment.

Sara went to the pharmacy and filled her prescriptions. She stared at the bottles and wondered how she got there. What would these medications do? How would they help manage her symptoms?

Parkinson's medications can help control symptoms including tremors, walking and problems with movement. These medications increase or substitute for dopamine as this is the chemical deficient in the brain of people with Parkinson's. One of the most prescribed drugs for Parkinson's is Carbidopa-levodopa® (generic names include Rytary®, Sinemet®, Duopa®), Levodopa is a natural chemical that passes into your brain and converts to dopamine. It is particularly important that you take your Parkinson's medications at the same time every day. If you don't take your medicines on time, you will notice your symptoms worsen making it hard to move around.

Are you having a tough time swallowing your medications? Try mixing it in with a spoonful of applesauce or pudding to help them go down smoother! Looking downwards while you swallow will also help you get down those pills easier. Set an alarm on your phone, smart home device or computer to remind you to take your medications on time. Use pill boxes and sort your morning and evening medications at the beginning of each week.

Talking pill bottles® are now available and they verbally can let you know information about your medication. Your pharmacist can record the name of the medication, the dosage, and when it is due into the cap. Whenever you need a reminder, all you need to do is push the button and this information can be repeated back to you. You can also ask your pharmacist for non-childproof bottles with easy open caps.

Why is timing of Parkinson's medication so important? If a person with Parkinson's disease does not receive their medication in time, it can make the symptoms worse—more tremors, increased rigidity, loss of balance, confusion and difficulty communicating, and it may take a longer time to recover ("off time").

Have your ever felt like you have times that you perform very well soon after you have taken your Parkinson's medications, and then you can feel that drug wearing off and your performance is not so great anymore? Well, you are not alone. There is commonly a peak performance period or" on time" and you can transfer better, walk better and move better. The period when the medications start to wear off and you feel your symptoms worsen is known as "off times."

It may occur in the morning, before the first dose of the medication or during the day between scheduled doses of your medications.

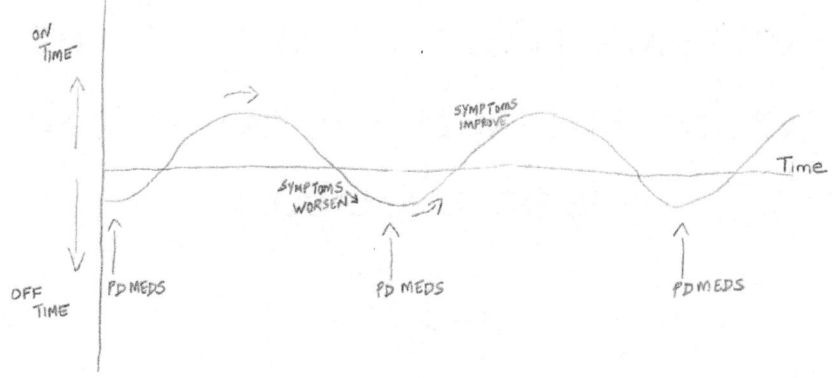

Figure 3a-Parkinson's medication-on and off times

Therefore, timing of Parkinson's medications is particularly important and it ensures there is a constant supply of dopamine in your system. Keep a journal and write down every time you have taken your medication. Use a pill box with sections for each day and time. Set alarms so that it can remind you when it is time for your next dose. Be vigilant of taking your medications timely, it will help you in the long run.

Take your medications on time, every time!

Chapter 4

My Brain Is Giving My Body the Wrong Messages and Making My World Smaller

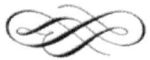

Sara had the official diagnosis now—Parkinson's. She started searching the Internet to find out all she could about this disease and how her brain was or was not working the way it should. Sara read up about how a Parkinson's brain gives the muscles the wrong smaller message and does not self-correct when undershooting a target leading to smaller movements. Wow, this started to make sense! Sara started to put the pieces together—the small steps, the small handwriting, the softer voice—all of this was because the brain was giving smaller messages to her body using network connections in the brain called neural pathways.

Going back to that chemical dopamine again, dopamine controls movement, with Parkinson's dopamine is less. So, that neural pathway in the brain that is used every day is giving a weaker signal to the muscles resulting in a smaller movement. Remember the example given earlier about a person with Parkinson's reaching for their phone, but their brain is telling them that they can stop reaching even before they have reached the needed distance to grasp the phone, undershooting the target? So, what could Sara do now? The neural pathway she had in her brain was giving her the wrong message. Well, no need to fear! The brain is an amazing organ, it can re-wire itself, a principle called neuroplasticity and new neural connections can be created. So, if your brain is giving you the wrong message and asking you to do things small, what can you do? Do the opposite, do things bigger! The brain is so used to using the small neural pathway day in and day out, it has been using this small pathway since you were diagnosed with Parkinson's. Not anymore! We need to create a new large pathway and retrain the brain to use this large neural pathway every time instead of that small one!

Have you ever been in your car, driving to work in the morning and suddenly you are there? You did not need to think about the stop signs and where to turn—your brain just knew because it has been doing this route every morning and it didn't require you to overthink it. Now, looking back to your first day at the job, you may have required the use of a navigation system that told you where to go.

That route to work was stored in your brain as a neural pathway and every morning after that, as you drove to work it got stronger and stronger and one day it was strong enough that you didn't even need to think about it—you got into your car, that neural pathway got activated and lit up and bam you're at work! Let us call this strong pathway Hulk.

Now suppose construction was to start on the highway that you use to get to work. You now need to use the local roads to get to work. So instead of turning right at your first stop, you need to make a left. First day of construction, you paid attention to the directions and made a left to get to the local roads. A new neural pathway in your brain has been formed—but since you only used it once, it is a weak pathway. Let us call this weak pathway Parker.

Now, on the second day of construction, you are running late to work, you do not have time to think, and you automatically hang a right at that first stop and get stuck in traffic. What happened? Your brain was on autopilot and was so used to using that strong neural pathway, Hulk, as it did every morning—it did not get time to think about the construction and that it needed to use the weak pathway, Parker, that was just created yesterday which resulted in you getting stuck in traffic.

The more and more you use that new pathway, Parker, as you drive to work using the new route, the stronger and stronger that pathway becomes. Until one day, it is as strong as the original strong pathway, Hulk, and you will not have to think about turning left to avoid construction, you will automatically do it.

This same concept applies to the brain of a person with Parkinson's. We can't use the small pathway that is giving your muscles the wrong messages anymore. Your brain will want to autopilot and use that small pathway, but we cannot allow that. That new stronger pathway needs to be created—a pathway that does things bigger and better! The more and more we think about using larger movements, the more that new large pathway lights up until one day, you don't have to think about it anymore and that will be the automatic pathway your brain decides to use.

Another comparison I like to use is comparing the brain of a person with Parkinson's to the dial of a radio. To hear the music, you need to turn the dial to the correct frequency and only then will you receive a clear signal. If the radio is not tuned in properly, all you can hear is scattered static noise. Well, in the brain of a person with Parkinson's this is what they hear all day long- scattered messages making the muscles perform smaller, inefficient movements. For the correct frequency to be tuned in, they must perform larger movements resulting in a clear message to the muscles to perform an efficient movement.

Your brain automatically tells you to do things smaller. Do the opposite, do things larger and create that new neural pathway to help manage your symptoms!

Chapter 5
I Am Losing My Voice

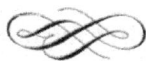

Sara was sitting in her living room watching her favorite TV show when she suddenly heard the phone ring. Sara answered the phone, it was her best friend Eva on the other line. "Hi Eva," Sara said softly. "Hello, Sara can you hear me? Hello? Can you speak up? I can't hear you; can you speak up Sara? There must be a bad connection." Sara knew deep down that it was not a connection issue, this wasn't the first time someone had told her to speak up, she realized her voice was becoming softer and harder to understand with each passing day. All she wanted was for her friends to understand what she was saying.

As a physical therapist, one thing I have heard patients with Parkinson's say a lot is that they feel they cannot speak as loud, and they have gotten quieter. I remember a patient that I had several years ago. when I was doing her evaluation, she became teary-eyed and said, "I used to be a talker, I could carry on conversations forever. But now I talk less because no one can hear me when I talk."

When carrying on a conversation, does it often occur that the other party can't hear you or they can't make out what you are trying to say? Do your spouse or your friends constantly ask you to repeat yourself because they couldn't hear you the first time? Sounds familiar, doesn't it?

Loss of voice is a common symptom of Parkinson's disease. A low, soft voice which is common in Parkinson's makes communication difficult leading to people having a challenging time understanding what you are saying. Well, why does it happen? Voice is controlled by the vocal cords and other muscles. The vocal cords are two bands of smooth muscle tissue found in the larynx (voice box). How does the sound of your voice generate? The first step is the vibration of your vocal cords anytime air passes through them from your lungs. But remember how we said that with Parkinson's the brain is giving a smaller message to the muscles because of that decrease in dopamine? Bingo! That's the reason the vocal cords vibrate smaller than needed producing a lower quality voice.

Don't lose hope! You can find your voice back! Create that new neural pathway in your brain to speak louder. When you are talking with your friends and family, shout out your words. Research has shown that speaking louder can help patients with Parkinson's communicate better. A speech-language pathologist will be able to help you with tips on how to speak louder. Exaggerate your pronunciation of words. Concentrate on using your tongue, lips, and jaw to enunciate each word loudly.

There are also apps available to work on improving loudness and quality of voice. Some of these apps are Speak Up for Parkinson's® and the Loud and Clear App® (available for iPad and smartphones). These apps are helpful as they are interactive, have visual and auditory feedback and a target for loudness. Audio-visual feedback is important because when seeing oneself and one's results, it provides an opportunity for self-analysis and setting goals and achievable targets for improvement. If you are a caregiver, avoid finishing sentences for someone with Parkinson's. Encourage them to try again and to talk louder this time. All they need most of the time is reminders to speak louder. LSVT LOUD® is an evidence-based treatment used by Speech Therapists to improve the vocal quality and loudness of voice for people with Parkinson's. I highly recommend this program.

Try to incorporate speaking loudly with everyday activities. I like to tell my patients, "If you aren't shouting, you aren't loud enough." You may not realize that you are speaking with a soft voice but hearing a voice recording of yourself may shock you. Remember, it is not your fault that your voice quality is low, it's the brain giving your vocal cords the wrong message making them vibrate smaller. Make those vocal cords vibrate bigger by shouting your words—this will seem awkward to you but trust me the words that come out will be at normal volume. Try to hold a note for as loud and as for long as you can. For example, try saying B for as loud and for as long as you can: "BEEEEEEEEEEEEEEEEEEEEEEEEEEEEEE." Time yourself and try it again but shoot for a longer hold each time. This will cause those vocal cords to vibrate and get stronger. Repeat, repeat, repeat for each letter of the alphabet! Do not let your voice prevent you from communicating and participating in social activities, speak louder!

Another tip I give my patients is to incorporate counting out loud while doing their daily exercises. "Come on, let's count out loud, 1,2,3..." as they do repetitions. The more frequently they speak louder, the more the brain will remember to do that with day-to-day conversations. Another way to build up the muscles that push air out of the lungs is by using a device called The Breather®. Using it daily can help with more syllables per breath and a stronger voice for people with Parkinson's. Read a book or newspaper as loud as you can, sing loudly and use a mirror to practice smiling big or frowning big to work on the muscles near your mouth.

In the later stages of the disease, speech amplifiers can be helpful to those who have a weak voice, throat or paralyzed vocal cords. The amplifier will increase the volume of spoken words Some even come with handheld or headset microphones. You can close your eyes if you get distracted while talking. This will reduce outside environmental distractions and help you focus on finding your voice. Do not get frustrated if you can't get the words out. Try breathing and counting to ten to help ease your mind and recollect your thoughts. Start speaking again with a loud voice to make it easier to communicate.

Have you ever tried to sing your words? It works wonders in getting the sentences out in people with Parkinson's who have a challenging time expressing themselves because the words aren't coming out.

You have power over your voice, be loud and claim it back!

Chapter 5: I Am Losing My Voice

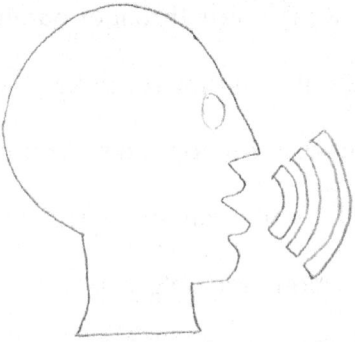

Figure 5a- Talk Louder

Chapter 6
My Handwriting is Getting Smaller

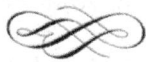

Sara's granddaughter's birthday was just around the corner. She goes to her den and wants to gift her with something special that she can cherish forever. 'Why not write a poem for little Elena?' she thinks to herself. She grabs a notepad and pen and starts writing down her thoughts, her memories of holding her when she was born and how proud she was of the beautiful little girl she was becoming. Sara looks at her notes and her heart becomes heavy. What happened to the beautiful handwriting that she once had? Her words were all cramped up and she couldn't make out the small handwriting and notes she had just jotted down.

One of the hallmark features of the onset of Parkinson's is smaller, cramped handwriting- micrographia. So why is handwriting affected in Parkinson's? You guessed it! Less dopamine = weaker signal from brain to hand muscles = less quality movement = small handwriting. Small, cramped handwriting is usually one of the first signs that patients notice. As the disease progresses, the handwriting usually gets worse and becomes even smaller.

Is there something that can be done to help manage this symptom of small handwriting? Of course, there is! Write big and activate that new large neural pathway in your brain we created!! I have my patients practice writing huge on double lines. The use of visual markers helps promote handwriting. My recommendation is to buy a wide-ruled notebook. Now, every day you will need to practice writing big—utilize two rows to write each word big and huge. Some patients like printing their name big, repeatedly. This will translate into getting their signature bigger and more legible. Other patients prefer to copy a novel into a notebook and to write each word big utilizing two rows. Lined paper also helps because it helps to keep the letters the same size. Regular training will strengthen the new big neural pathway we are creating. Practicing handwriting helps Parkinson's brains to discover new nerve cell connections in the areas of the brain responsible for vision and movement learning. Writing in print versus writing in cursive will force you to slow down and try to form each letter making them bigger and more legible. The more you practice overexaggerating the size of your handwriting, the more legible and normal sized it will become!

I remember a patient that I was treating for Parkinson's several years ago. This patient had micrographia and their handwriting became progressively smaller and illegible over the years. His main goal was to be able to write a check that was legible. For his treatment, I printed a bunch of blank check templates and had him write checks out for his electric bills, water bills and phone bills. And then I had him do that again and again, each time making sure that he practiced writing them big. We continued to practice every day until one day his wife came up to me and exclaimed, "I can read his handwriting! He can help with the bills again!"

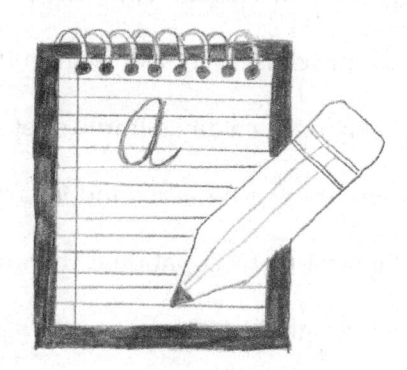

Figure 6a- Practice writing bigger

Surprisingly, another trick to get the handwriting bigger is closing your eyes while writing. Taking away the visual feedback that is normally present helps patients to concentrate on one less thing and improve legibility of handwriting. Amazing, isn't it?

There are many tools that can help make writing easier. Pen grips, which are round or triangular rubber or foam cylinders can make it easier to grip or hold a pen or pencil. Find pens that are larger so that they are easier to grip and stabilize. You can also add a few rubber bands to your existing pens to make them larger and easier to grip. Weighted pens are beneficial for people who have tremors in their hands.

Strengthening the muscles in your hands and fingers is also important. You can purchase Play-Doh® from the store and practice squeezing it and relaxing each day. Simple stretches like opening and closing your fingers or creating a fist and squeezing your hand will help. See your Physical or Occupational therapist for specific hand exercises that may be right for you.

Write and write until you get a surprising result in your handwriting!

Chapter 7

It's So Hard to Roll and Move Around in Bed

The lights are out, and Sara lay in bed thinking about her day. Her back is hurting and so she decides to lay on her side. She tries and tries, but she feels stuck, her muscles feel stiff, and she feels frozen in bed.

Have you been having difficulty getting out of bed? Do you often feel stuck? Do your muscles feel stiff when you wake up in the morning? These features are quite common in patients with Parkinson's. So, what can you do?

Stretching for a few minutes while in bed helps loosen your muscles making it easier to move around. Reach your hand overhead as far as they can go in a quick big movement, hold it at the end range for five to ten seconds and then bring it back down. Repeat this for ten repetitions, each one bigger than the one before.

Several of my patients report taking forever to get out of bed. What can help with this? Overreach while you roll! Instead of just reaching for the end of the bed or the bedrail if you have one, reach for the wall. Turn with a big, intense movement. The bigger you roll, the easier it will be to get out of bed. Once you have rolled with a big movement, it is time for you to push off and sit at the edge of the bed. When you are doing this, push off the bed as if you are angry with it—that will make the movement more intense, resulting in an easier transition to the side of the bed.

Practice this over and over again—moving around in bed, — starting with rolling, to pushing off and sitting at the edge of the bed. The brain can re-wire itself- one of the driving forces to making the brain change (neuroplasticity) is repeating a movement often so that the brain remembers that movement pattern the next time it is attempted. Another main principle for brain change is that the movement needs to be intense. So, practice getting out of bed with a large intense movement and the brain will remember to do this each time leading to a more efficient way of getting up.

Leg lifters are a piece of adaptive equipment that can be looped around the leg and assist a person to lift their leg into or out of bed. It is lightweight and easy to use and can help you with your independence getting in or out of bed.

In the later stages of the disease, it may become difficult for a person with Parkinson's to roll in bed. If you are a caregiver, it is advised to create a drawsheet by folding a flat sheet into a large rectangle and placing it on top of the fitted sheet from the chest to the thighs. When you need to roll your loved one towards you, grasp the two ends of the folded sheet furthest from you, then with your palms up move the draw sheet towards you. Make sure to keep your knees slightly bent so that they can help with the pull and keep you from hurting your back. If the bed can be raised, bring it up so that your back is protected.

Chapter 8

I'm Stuck, and I Can't Stand Up

~~~~~

Sara's grandson Jaden comes to pick her up and take her out to lunch. Sara is hesitant to go as she tries to avoid public places as much as she can ever since her diagnosis. Thoughts started to cross Sara's mind. 'What will others think when they see me move? Will I embarrass myself in front of others?' Sara hesitantly gets into the car and Jaden drives them to a fancy restaurant. He opens the car door for grandma to get out, but Sara can't get up—she feels stuck to the car seat and isn't able to move.

Feeling stuck and having a hard time standing up is very common with Parkinson's disease.

There are several steps required for the simple movement of standing up. Look at all the below steps.

- Scoot to the edge of the chair.
- Make sure that your feet are behind you.
- Hold on to the armrests of your chair.
- You are going to try to lean all the way forward, "nose over toes."
- Let's rock forward and then on the count of three we will stand up.
- 1, 2, 3 ok, stand!
- Come taller, taller.
- Tuck that bottom in.
- Ok good, you are standing.

See how many steps are involved with just standing up? Now with Parkinson's we do not want to complicate things, we want to keep everything as simple as possible. It gets harder and harder for a person with Parkinson's to concentrate on multiple things, and harder to multitask. So, can you imagine how difficult it is to do the simple movement of standing up? Now, seeing all the steps involved, it is not so simple anymore, is it?

How can we make this now complex movement of standing up simpler? Easy! Just one simple command, "Stand up big and reach for the ceiling!" Remember with Parkinson's, the brain gives the muscles the wrong message to do things smaller. And so, when they try to stand up, they automatically want to use that bad pathway and hence the movement is smaller, and they feel stuck and cannot complete the movement.

When my patients feel like they are getting stuck, I tell them not to get frustrated, instead just stop, reset, and stand up with a large movement. I sometimes have them reach for the ceilings with their arms while they stand in a big movement to assist with that elongation of the body and to get them standing taller. The bigger the stand, the more efficient the movement.

Standing up taller requires practice as it does not come naturally, especially for a person with Parkinson's. Daily practice of standing up tall with multiple repetitions is needed to get the brain to use that big pathway each time you stand up.

Stand up tall and reach for the starts! The sky is the limit!

CHAPTER 8: I'M STUCK, AND I CAN'T STAND UP

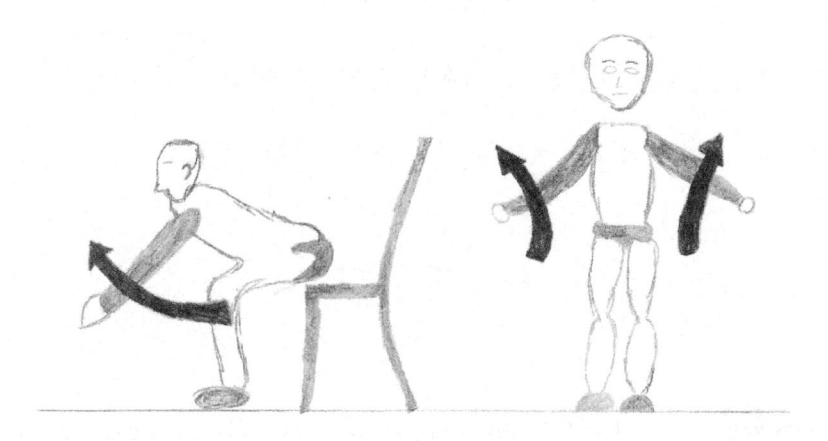

Figure 8 a- Practice standing up with a one large movement

Chapter 9

My Steps are Smaller, and I Shuffle Them When I Walk

Every Tuesday afternoon, Sara's friends would meet up at the community park to exercise and walk the trails. It is a beautiful day, the sky is blue, and the birds are singing, what a wonderful day for a walk! But all Sara could think of was how difficult it was getting for her to keep up with her friends. Sara noticed that her steps were smaller and that sometimes they would run together making her feel like she was going to fall forward, her arm stiffly next to her side as though she was wearing a cast and barely swinging while walking. She didn't want to burden her friends or slow them down, so she canceled on them and decided to stay at home.

When you visit with your neurologist, one of the things they usually have you do is walk while they observe. What are they looking for while you walk? Small, shuffled steps with decreased use of your arms while you walk are common characteristics in Parkinson's. You guessed it! The brain gave those muscles in your legs and arms the wrong message resulting in smaller steps and stiffer movements.

So, what can you do? Take huge, giant steps! I tell my patients they need to take Pink Panther steps, as big as they can get them. Swing those arms! This will feel awkward, but that's ok—we need to get the brain trained in doing things bigger instead of smaller, and the only way to do that is to incorporate largeness into every activity—even walking. Many times, patients have what we call a festinating gait pattern—they feel like their steps run all together and they feel like they are falling forward while walking. If this is happening, remind yourself to stop when it happens, think about doing it larger, then resume your walking, starting with a big step.

Practice taking big steps forwards, backwards, and sideways while you are at home. The bigger they are, the better. Put markers on the ground to set a target on how big you want your step to be each time you practice, having a visual goal can keep those steps big each time. When walking, try to shout out, "left, right, left, right" with each step—it will remind you to keep the steps large and help you concentrate on your movements. Practice in front of a mirror and pretend like you are marching high with each step. Swing your opposite arm when taking a step to improve the rhythm of your walking and it helps to reduce the body weight from your legs which lessens fatigue and loosens up your arms and shoulders.

What is freezing in Parkinson's? It is the momentary paralysis of movement due to Parkinson's—you will feel like your foot is stuck to the ground and cannot move. Freezing typically occurs with an inability to take a first step. However, once that first step is taken, they can continue walking. Why does this happen? The brain has separate motor control pathways for initiating walking and another one for maintaining walking. So, the first pathway for initiating walking is affected with Parkinson's resulting in feeling stuck to the ground, but the second pathway of maintenance of walking is not affected that much. Once that first step is taken, walking resumes with the second pathway that maintains walking and it lights up and takes control. So, what can you do to overcome the difficulty of initiating that first step which causes the feeling of being stuck to the ground? Usually, you do not have to think about taking that first step or think about swinging your arms when you walk, this is an unconscious automatic activity. However, for patients with Parkinson's it is not automatic, and the unconscious brain circuit is not working. So, instead, use the conscious brain circuit that is still working! Anytime you feel stuck, stop, and give time for your brain to reset. Now, think about a different leg movement like marching or swinging the leg forward to unfreeze that first step. Afterward, the pathway in the brain that maintains walking will take over.

I have found music with beats during walking extremely helpful in getting the steps more equal and coordinated with each beat they hear. Walk to a regular beat to help prevent freezing. There are also apps available for metronomes, like Beats Medical Parkinson's app®, that will provide an auditory cue each time they are to take a big step. This has been found to be an amazingly effective method to remind people with Parkinson's to take big, equal, coordinated steps. Music not only helps smooth and symmetrical walking, but also assists with decreasing facial masking, promoting better movement of the arms and legs, and improving loudness and quality of voice. Another way to overcome freezing is to find a target on the floor and step on it. You can also use a laser beam one to two feet ahead of you on the floor and think about stepping on that target spot with each step.

Have you ever felt like you get stuck in the doorways or near thresholds, or have you felt like you feel frozen and cannot move in tight spaces and corners? What can you do to overcome this? That's right, stop—reset your brain—resume movement with a big step. The reason you need to stop is that your brain is giving your muscles the wrong message again, so you need to stop so that the brain can reset and use the big pathway. The next time you are stuck at that doorway or threshold, don't overthink it; just stop, and then take your next step big and huge. Even in corners, take wide big turns. If you are experiencing freezing, using a cane with a small ball protrusion at the bottom can help trick your mind into thinking that you are stepping over something. If you feel like your foot is glued to the ground, imagine that you are about to march and pick up that leg and bang it back on the ground as if you are squishing ants on the floor with your foot! Retrain that brain and repeat, repeat, repeat! The more you practice these difficult movements, the stronger that new pathway becomes, and it will help you overcome your obstacles!

If you wear bifocals, stairs can be a challenge because it throws off your depth perception especially while going down the stairs. Sometimes placing a neon tape at the edge of each step will help identify where each step is ending and assist with that depth perception. If you have one leg that is stronger than the other, it is best to go up the stairs one step at a time, leading with your strong leg. When you go down the stairs, go down with your weaker or less stiff leg. A good mnemonic for remembering this is "Good people go to heaven; bad people go you know where"—always lead with the good and come down with the bad.

If you need a wheelchair, consider buying one that is lightweight so that it can be easily folded and transported in your car. Always ask your car manufacturer if they offer discounts or rebates for the purchase of adaptive equipment for people with disabilities. You may also want to investigate getting a wheelchair cushion to protect your skin from pressure injury. For anyone who may need a wheelchair, it is important to relieve pressure off your bottom by doing mini pushups from the wheelchair periodically.

If you need a walker, my recommendation is to get a U-step walker®. The U-step walker® particularly helps Parkinson's patients regain their stability while walking. It has a very stable U-shaped base that prevents it from wiggling when walking, making it feel more secure and it braces you in every direction, which prevents falls. The U-step walker® can also be used in narrow and tight indoor spaces. The braking mechanism helps you stand up from any seated position. The brake mechanism is opposite that of a normal rollator. In a U-step walker, for the walker to move the handles need to be gripped, and when you need to stop the walker you release the grip, giving you more control especially when you feel like your steps are about to run together (festinating gait). This reverse brake mechanism is especially useful in patients with Parkinson's. Additional accessories including a laser light that gives a visual cue on increasing step length can be purchased. There are also some canes also available with laser light technology.

The mind is a powerful thing, get control of your life and do things bigger!

Chapter 10

Dressing Myself and Combing My Hair is Taking Longer Than It Should

---

Sara just finished taking a calm, relaxing, soothing shower. She stares at the clothes that she laid on the bed. She shakes her head knowing that what used to be a simple task was now something she dreaded to do. This simple task used to take only a few minutes, and now it took much longer. She decides to comb her hair first. She reaches for the brush, and finally grasps it slowly. Her long black curls are waiting to be combed, but this too is not an easy task. She starts from the top but stops mid-way and is stuck. 'Why does everything have to be so hard,' she thinks to herself.

Is it taking you a long time to get dressed in the morning? Are you not able to pull your shirt over your head? Is it getting harder to do buttons?

Smaller movements can lead to taking longer to perform normal day-to-day activities like getting dressed and combing your hair. The main tip I'm going to give you again is to do this larger. How can you comb your hair larger you may ask. Well start from the top and comb it straight down with a quick movement—overshot aiming the brush to your waist and not stopping at your shoulder. If you aim for a further distance, your movement will end up where it should. When putting on your t-shirt in the morning, open the hole for your head wide open and with an intense large movement, place it over your head. Next, grab one sleeve of the T-shirt and shove your hand through in a punching movement. Repeat for the other sleeve. Now, grab both ends of the T-shirt and with one large intense movement, pull it down fast, aiming for your feet. Even though you aimed for your feet, the shirt ended up right at your waist like it should be.

Make sure to be sitting down while performing dressing tasks, especially if your balance is unsteady. If you have one arm or leg that is stiffer than the other, put this limb into the sleeve or pant leg first. Do a few stretching exercises before starting dressing activities. Dressing will be easier when your medications are working, so plan to dress during your "on time." It is good practice to set out your clothes the night before. Try to buy clothing one size larger than you normally wear. Choose clothing with elastic waistbands or Velcro closures. If you have one side that is stiffer because of Parkinson's, then always dress your weaker or stiffer limb first. To undress, do the opposite—take the clothes off the stronger side first. Visual biofeedback goes a long way in dressing with Parkinson's. Dress in front of a mirror to help find the sleeves and watch yourself utilizing big movements as you dress.

Do you love wearing your buttoned shirts but are having a tough time with the buttons because of your tremors? Here is a trick for you. Shake your hands for ten seconds and try the button again, the tremors should temporarily stop. If it tremors return, repeat. Instead of shaking your hands, you could also clap your hands ten times and then try again. Even stretching your hands and arms out in front of you has shown to reduce tremors temporarily. Another trick with buttons is to pretend you are angry and then try doing the buttons, the energy and intensity built up from the feeling of anger will help improve the quality of the movement and take less time to perform. There is also a tool called a button hook that can assist with buttoning shirts. You can also sew buttons on with an elastic thread which will provide more space for the button to go through.

What about pants? After you go to the bathroom—do you have a tough time pulling up your pants? What should you do? That's right—do it bigger! Grab onto both sides of your pants and get a good grip—now, real hard pull up aiming for the ceiling. Your pants will end up right at the waist where they need to be if you aim for the ceiling. Over-exaggerated movements will equal to normal size movements when performing activities of daily living.

How about socks? Same thing—big intense movement and your socks should get easier to put on. Hold on to either side of the sock and pull up with one large, intense movement. There is also a tool available to help get socks on called a sock aid. Once you apply the sock to the sock aid, pull with a big intense movement to get your socks on easier.

Are your shoelaces getting harder to tie? Remove your shoelaces and get elastic shoelaces applied instead. They are available to purchase through Amazon and your shoes will be converted to easy slip-ons. Sometimes switching to Velcro shoes is advised as they are easier to slip on and off. Even with Velcro shoes, make sure to pull that Velcro off with a big, intense, fast movement so that it doesn't take forever to put on or take off.

Sit while you do your hair, shave, or apply makeup. Use an electric toothbrush for brushing your teeth—they have longer handles that are easier to grasp. Use an electric razor especially if you experience tremors. Electric razors are easier to hold and require fewer fine motor skills to use. Switch to using pump-type containers for your soaps and lotions. It is much easier to pump than to squeeze a bottle for a person with Parkinson's.

If you are freezing during self-care activities, there are things that you can do to break the freezing episode. So, if a freezing episode comes along while you are putting on your shirt, stop first to reset your brain. Next, try to count out loud or try using a metronome or even turn on some music. That usually does the trick.

If you are a caregiver, make sure to keep positive and be encouraging. Allow the person with Parkinson's to do as much for themselves as possible. Remove that tendency to jump in and help with a task because you can do it faster. This not only decreases their confidence, but also enables them to depend on you in the future for these tasks. If they use the right tips and strategies and perform every task with a big effort, you will be surprised to see how much they can do for themselves! Provide cues as necessary. Patients with Parkinson's perform better with external cues and visual feedback. Their automatic internal cueing system is affected, so provide the external cues- the reminders for bigger movements. For example, if they have a mirror in front of them as they dress, they can self-correct when the movements are not big enough (visual cues) and you can provide the reminders as needed to perform the movements bigger (external cues).

There are some adaptive tools that can also help with dressing tasks such as zipper pulls, reachers, dressing sticks, Velcro, sock aides, and long shoehorns. Your Occupational Therapist can show you how to use these tools to improve your independence.

CHAPTER 10: DRESSING MYSELF AND COMBING MY HAIR IS TAKING LONGER THAN IT SHOULD

Live life independently again!

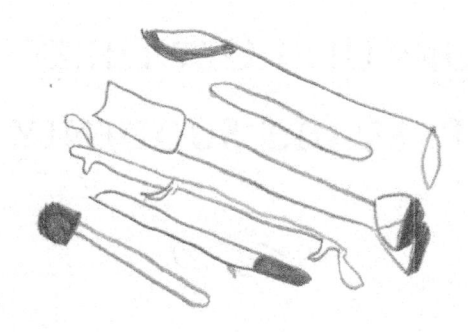

Figure 10a- Commonly used adaptive equipment

Chapter 11
When I Get Up, I Get Dizzy, and My Blood Pressure Suddenly Drops

Sara is in bed, all wrapped up in her comfy new blanket, not a bother in the world. "Ding dong", the doorbell rings and Sara knows it's her long-awaited package from Amazon. She's excited to see the beautiful dress she ordered and suddenly tries to get up. Whoa! Her head is spinning, and she feels faint. These dizzy spells have been happening more often lately.

If you are experiencing light-headedness with positional changes like lying down to standing, it may be because your blood pressure dropped- a term known as orthostatic hypotension. Blood pressure variations including orthostatic hypotension is common in people with Parkinson's. Common symptoms of low blood pressure include dizziness or feeling lightheaded, fainting, or passing out, confusion or trouble concentrating, fatigue or weakness, nausea, or vomiting, blurred or distorted vision, fast or shallow breathing and agitation. If you think you are experiencing this, make sure to call your doctor so that you can be evaluated. If you have a blood pressure cuff, you can check your blood pressure in various positions and see if there are variations. First, check your blood pressure while laying down. Next, check it when sitting at the edge of the bed. Last, check it while standing. Invest in purchasing a blood pressure cuff, it will come in handy.

Sometimes all it takes for symptoms to resolve is to sit on the edge of your bed for a minute or steadying yourself for a moment when you stand up. If you feel faint while exercising, have someone check your blood pressure and pulse. If your systolic blood pressure or the upper number is less than ninety, it means your blood pressure has dropped. Do not continue exercising if you are feeling faint, stop and take a break.

Another way to treat orthostatic hypotension is to decrease the pooling of blood in your legs with the use of compression stockings. How do they work? The compression stockings (also known as Ted hose) will compress the veins in your legs, which, in turn, help reduce swelling and increase blood flow. These stockings should be worn when you are up and about; they need to be taken off when you are in bed. It is recommended that they are applied first thing in the morning, and you must make sure that they are not rolled or bunched up, which may lead to decreased circulation.

Abdominal binders are also used to help improve blood pressure. This is a compression garment that is worn around the waist to help prevent blood pooling and thus helps improve blood pressure.

If you are symptomatic and your blood pressure is low, it is good to know a recovery position that will help increase your blood pressure. The best position for increasing blood pressure is one in which the head is low, and the body and legs are elevated using pillows or an inclined surface. When a person is placed in this position, gravity pulls the blood down towards the vital organs of the brain and heart. This pulling of blood results in increased blood volume and increased cardiac output and in return increases the blood pressure.

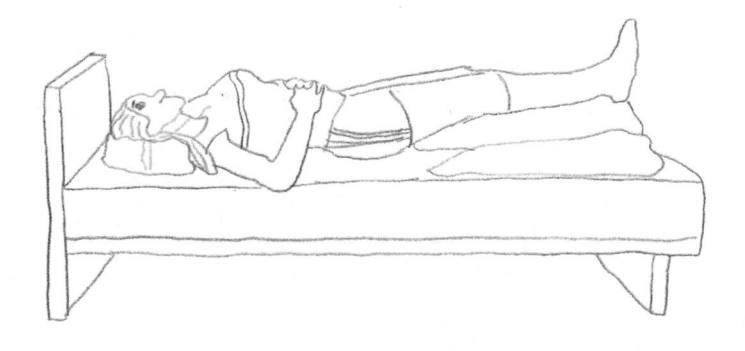

Figure 11a- Recovery position for low blood pressure

Dehydration is another cause for orthostatic hypotension. Make sure to drink plenty of fluids to avoid a drop in your blood pressure. Adding a lemon wedge to your water can make it more flavorful and appealing. Try purchasing a water bottle that keeps the water cold and can keep track of how much water you drink in a day. Drink water before, during and after a workout to keep hydrated.

If symptoms of light-headedness are more pronounced and you feel off balance like you are going to fall, your doctor will look at your medications and may make some adjustments. Your doctor may prescribe medications such as Midodrine®, droxidopa®, fludrocortisone® or pyridostigmine® to help treat the low blood pressure.

Chapter 12

My Tremors Make It Hard for Me to Eat with a Spoon

※

It is Thanksgiving and all of Sara's family and friends are here to celebrate. There's Ninan peeking into the oven checking on his green bean casserole, there's Suja, Sunil and Philip setting the table. Sara looks around and smiles seeing her grandsons- Jeremy, Jalen and Jaden all joking with each other. Her little granddaughters Elena, Naomi, and Sarina all decked up with new nail polish, managing to put a discreet layer of makeup on their faces without their parents knowing. "It's time to eat!." exclaims Susan—Sara's sister-in-law. Sara's joy became fear. She felt that pit in her stomach, she was anxious and afraid that everyone would see how sloppy she was when she ate. The tremors made it extremely hard for her to bring her food to her mouth without it spilling.

When you eat, does your food end up all over you because of your tremors? Do not worry—you are not alone. Tremors are very common in Parkinson's disease, and it occurs due to the lower levels of dopamine in your brain, which causes problems with movement. It commonly occurs with rest. More than seventy-five percent of PD patients experience resting tremors at some point during the disease process.

The "pill-rolling tremor" usually refers to tremors of the fingers (usually the thumb plus the other fingers), that makes it look like the person is rolling a pill between their fingers. This is most often the part of the body where tremors start. The tremors usually lessen during sleep or when the body part is actively in use. For example, your hand may shake while sitting, but when you reach out to shake hands with someone, it may go away.

Although tremors are most seen in the hands, they can occur in other parts of the body including the legs, jaws, or lips. This can interfere with everyday activities like eating, dressing, shaving, writing and other activities of daily living. Tremors may start by affecting only one side of the body but as the disease progresses, it can develop on both sides.

If you have tremors or a weak grip, make sure not to fill your cup to the brim—only fill it up half-full. You can wind some rubber bands around the glass for better grip. If needed, you can drink from a sports water bottle instead of a glass to prevent spills.

Some assistive devices that can be used to help control tremors during everyday activities are listed below and are available to purchase through Amazon or directly through the websites listed in the Resources section of this book.

- GYENNO Parkinson spoon and fork®: Although costly, this tool electronically stabilizes the attached utensil and controls the shaking up to eighty-five percent, which helps prevent spilling.
- Use a rocker knife instead of the traditional straight knife. The rocker knife utilizes a seesaw motion and uses less energy in comparison to the traditional knife.
- Weighted utensils: Weighted utensils like a weighted spoon, weighted fork or a weighted knife help to stabilize tremors. They are wider in circumference and can be easier to grip if you have Parkinson's.
- Plate guards are unique plates that prevents spills and promotes independence while minimizing messy spills at mealtime.

CHAPTER 12: MY TREMORS MAKE IT HARD FOR ME TO EAT WITH A SPOON

- Pace Dycem® rubber pads or Rubbermaid® mats underneath utensils like plates, cups and serving dishes to keep them from sliding.
- Weighted wide grip pens: Weighted pens provide stable writing for patients with Parkinson's and essential tremors.
- Hand weight ®: This weight can be placed on the back of your hand to help decrease tremors with activity and allows your fingers and hand to move more freely.
- Weighted cups and plates also help with controlling tremors while drinking or eating.
- Universal cuff utensil holders® can assist with stabilizing the weighted utensils during eating.

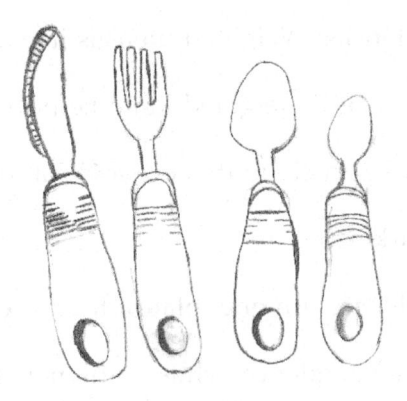

Figure 12a- Weighted utensils

Some helpful tips for eating include keeping your chin down as you chew and swallow and taking small bite-size portions with each bite. Make sure to chew thoroughly before swallowing to avoid pocketing of food in your mouth. After eating, it is important to rinse your mouth with antibacterial mouthwash. Pocketing of food is common with Parkinson's and residual food is often found in the mouth because of swallowing problems associated with Parkinson's. Residual food attracts harmful bacteria that can lead to poor oral health and infections and the bacteria can travel to your heart leading to damage there as well.

If you have problems with drooling, try to chew gum—it will help remind you to swallow more often. Try to make it a habit to swallow your saliva regularly—your brain is slowing down the salivary swallow response as well, and so reminding yourself to do this every so often will prevent you from drooling. Get confident with eating again!

Chapter 13

I Fall More Often Now

※

Sara was walking to the kitchen to prepare her morning coffee. Her foot caught the kitchen throw rug and she fell hard on her back. As she hit the ground with a "thud," at first, she was shocked, and disappointed in herself. Sara gazed up to the ceiling and never realized how cold the bare hardwood floor was. Tears started to flow in desperation as she continued to stare at the ceiling.

Balance problems are quite common in the Parkinson's population. It is normal to feel scared of falling, especially if you have fallen before. Even those who do not fall can develop the fear if they have a friend who's fallen. There are things that you can do to be less fearful of falling.

Fear may develop as people begin to lose control over their balance. Problems with vision, the inner ear, or the sense of touch in a person's feet and ankles can occur and can lead to altered balance which in turn can cause a fall. Some people tighten their muscles when they feel they are about to fall. This stiffening can limit the range of motion and make a fall more likely.

It is important to be able to reach for help in the unfortunate event that you have fallen. Always keep a cellphone with you. I tell my patients to put their cellphones in a lanyard around their necks while they move around so that they have it with them constantly throughout the day. Keep a list of emergency numbers near your phone. You can program your phone for the speed-dial features, or you can activate the voice control features on your phone. There are home monitoring devices also available. If you fall, you can press a button on the device around your neck or wrist. This alerts emergency responders to come and help you.

When you can, choose chairs with long armrests. There are handrails available to purchase for couches if that is where you usually sit during the day. Using rails or armrests improves safety when getting in and out of a chair. When sitting down, back up until you feel the chair against the back of both your legs. If you have a walker, back up with the walker. Next, reach back for the armrests and lean forward to sit down on the chair. If your couch is too low, making it hard to stand up, consider purchasing couch risers.

One easily overlooked safety tip is to keep things within reach. Walker trays are available for walkers to easily assist in carrying items or food from one room to another. Keep things you often use within reach including water, remote control, reading books or tissues. Keep items in the same place to establish a familiar routine. You can also use a tote bag strapped around your walker to carry commonly used items safely. Walker slides can be attached to the back legs of your walker to help with smooth, easy mobility with reduced noise in comparison with traditional walkers.

Some of the medications that you may be on can lead to side effects that lead to a fall. Common medications that can cause these side effects are blood pressure, pain medications, medications for sleep, and antidepressants. Review your medications with your doctor because the way your body reacts to medicines can change as you age. Your doctor will be able to make changes to your medications if needed.

Regular exercise and staying active are the best ways to prevent falls. Balance, strength, endurance, and flexibility all come from exercise. Good activities to improve balance include Tai chi, yoga, dance and stretching. Yoga and tai chi not only help with balance but also provide a time for recollection and quiet meditation. Cleansing your mind with these activities can help you focus on what's important in your life—your health and your family. Peer support has shown to be highly effective—get out and exercise with a group, it will build up your confidence so that you can actively work on your balance. Also remember to use the heel-toe walking method. Focus on getting the heel down first with every step. When you are walking, be aware of your surroundings.

Steps to get off the floor if you have fallen

If you have fallen, the first thing you need to do is make sure you are not hurt. Take a few minutes to make sure you are not in pain or suffering from any injuries. If you are hurt, wait for help before attempting to get up. It is important that you know how to get up safely if you are not hurt. Fall recovery is crucial to understand for anyone who has Parkinson's. The following are the steps to follow to get up from the floor after a fall.

1. Roll towards a sturdy chair or sofa.

Chapter 13: I Fall More Often Now

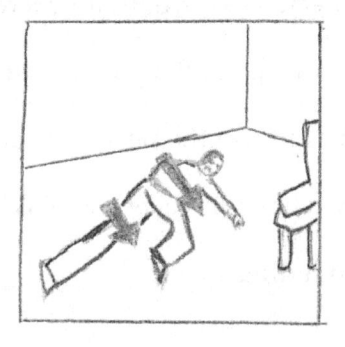

Figure 13a Roll

2. Push your upper body up and crawl towards the chair, try to put your hands on the chair

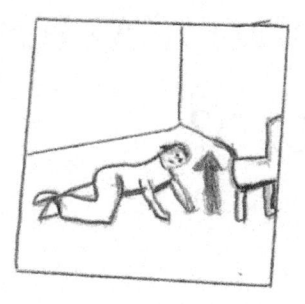

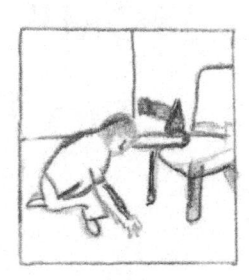

Figure 13b, and 13c- Push up, crawl to chair, hand on chair

3. Kneel with one leg forward and use your hands to slowly rise and turn your body to sit on the chair. Sit down and rest for a few minutes before trying to move.

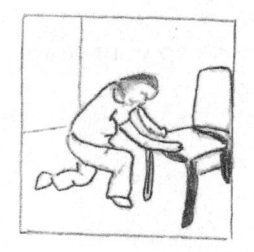

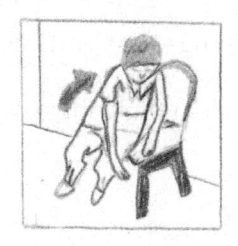

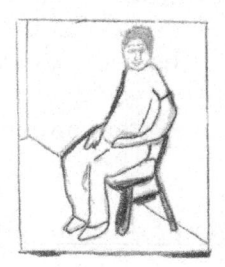

Figure 13d, 13e and 13f- Kneel, Rise-Turn to sit- Sit and recover

Chapter 14

What Home Modifications Do I Need?

Sara is at her friend Eva's house and notices some recent home improvements that were done. She sees a grab bar in the bathroom and notices the furniture re-arranged. Eva spots Sara looking around and lets her know how much the new modifications has helped her with her mobility and independence.

There are several things that you can do to keep your home safe, prevent falls and improve your independence.

General home safety

Removing loose carpets and rugs can also help prevent falls at home. Remove all throw rugs in your home; they are one of the common causes of falls in the elderly. Re-arrange furniture to open the area and remove unnecessary obstacles in your path. You can also keep the furniture in strategic locations in case you need to hold onto them as you walk. Remove things that can trip you like boxes or cords. Do not store items on stairs and keep walkways clear. Rearrange furniture in your home so that walkers or wheelchairs can easily maneuver around chairs, sofas, and tables. You can also install a railing along a long hallway in your home or in the bathroom to help with steadying yourself and for additional support. When installing railings, make sure that they are securely anchored to the studs in the wall. Keep electrical cords and telephone wires tucked away in corners to avoid them being a trip hazard.

Car:

When transferring in and out of a car, it is best to utilize the front passenger seat of your car. Make sure it is positioned in the furthest back position. Avoid vehicles that are too low, they will be difficult to get in and out of. You can purchase a portable car handle assist® to help you get in and out of your vehicle. It helps with providing stability and balance when standing or sitting in the car. This handle fits into the latch of your car door and makes for a steady surface to push off from without additional modifications needed to your car. Seatbelt extenders are available to improve grasp, pull and buckle up.

Lighting:

Improve lighting by adding night lights or adding in automatic lighting that illuminates with sunset will help in preventing falls during the middle of the night bathroom breaks. It is best to use the highest-wattage light bulbs available. You can replace traditional light switches with rocker-panel switches as they are easier to use for people with Parkinson's as they require less fine motor control. Motion detector light switches are also available for purchase at your hardware store. Nowadays, with advanced technology, you can utilize smart home speakers like Amazon echo® (Alexa) or Google mini® to help control lights, TVs, locks and much more. If you convert your thermostat to Nest®, you can control your home temperature from your Google mini® or through your smartphone.

Doorknobs

Regular doorknobs can be difficult to manipulate for a person with Parkinson's. Replace them with lever handles that are easier to grasp and use. If you cannot replace your doorknobs, consider wrapping a few rubber bands around them for better grip.

Bathroom

For your bathroom, add in safety grab bars near your toilet to assist with getting up off the toilet. When installing grab bars, make sure that they are securely anchored to the studs in the wall so they will be able to support your body weight. Add in a raised toilet seat or toilet safety frame to increase the height of your toilet thus producing in an easier stand. Invest in getting a bidet for your toilet. A bidet is a plumbing fixture that can help with toileting hygiene after urination or a bowel movement. Bidets can attach to your toilet and can be installed to the side of the toilet bowl with a detachable hose. A bidet can help anybody who has difficulty with reaching and wiping as there is less wrist action involved in cleaning hard to reach areas. Another tool that can help with wiping hard to reach areas is called a bottom buddy®. One end grips any tissue or toilet paper securely and releases the paper with the push of a button and it is an easy solution for cleanliness when reaching is difficult. Install a handheld shower in your shower to assist with cleaning hard-to-reach areas and for energy conservation. Install grab bars that are securely anchored in your shower as well to assist with stability. You may need to get a shower chair or a tub transfer bench to sit down safely while you shower. If needed, you can replace your glass shower door with a lightweight shower curtain for easier access to the shower. You can get a nonslip bathmat as well. Invest in a superior quality terry cotton robe that can be used right after your shower to help with quick drying and energy conservation. If your bathroom doorway is too narrow to accommodate your walker or wheelchair, you can remove the door and replace it with a black shower curtain liner for privacy. Store commonly used items like towels and washcloths at eye level to help avoid reaching and bending.

Doorways

Doorways should be at least thirty-two inches wide to allow for wheelchair access. You can install offset hinges that allow the door to swing out instead of in, which will increase the door opening by a few inches.

Steps and Ramps

If you have steps to enter your home, it is best to install hand railings on both sides of the steps to ease going up and coming down the stairs. If you have stairs within your home, rails on both sides are recommended. In later stages of the disease, it may become difficult to go up and down stairs within the home, especially if your bedroom is on the second floor. In these cases, consider installing a stairlift.

Stairlifts are installed on the wall of your stairway and allow the person to sit in a chair while the power lift takes you upstairs or downstairs with the push of a button. For thresholds or stairs, try using neon tape at the edge of each step to help identify where each step is ending. If a ramp is recommended at your entrance, make sure it is installed on a non-slip resistant surface and is one foot in length for every inch in vertical rise (maximum slope of eight feet, minimum width of forty-eight inches). Consider installing a ramp with a railing (handrails are required if slope is greater than five degrees).

Kitchen

In your kitchen, make sure that commonly used items are within reach, on the countertop or in a cabinet at eye level. You can place your utensils and plates in a drying rack near the sink to avoid having to constantly reach overhead to cabinets to retrieve these items. Avoid stacking or piling objects on top of each other. To make cleaning easier, purchase a broom with a long-handled dustpan. This allows you to sweep up dust while remaining in a standing position. Install pull-out shelves for your lower cabinets to reduce the need of bending over and straining your back. Consider soft close drawers which will reduce the chances of fingers getting accidentally caught when closing the drawer. Some cabinet lazy Susans can be installed to get you easy access to items in your cabinet that would have been otherwise hard to see or reach.

Bedroom

In your bedroom, consider repositioning your bed against the wall to make it more accessible. Make sure to keep your phone and other essentials within reach. Bed rails can be installed under the mattress that can help you move easier in bed and will come in handy when rolling and moving to the edge of your bed as you can use it for support. If your bed is too tall, consider replacing the box spring with a low profile one which will reduce the height of the bed by at least three inches. If you are planning to buy a new bed, invest in one where the head of the bed can be elevated. Wearing satin nightclothes can assist with moving around easier when in bed. If you have problems with incontinence at night, consider buying a plastic mattress cover and placing it under your fitted sheet. Adult incontinence briefs are also available for purchase to wear at night if needed.

Living Room

In your living room, it is best to get a chair that is sturdy and stable and has armrests. If you prefer to sit on your sofa but it is too low, you can purchase couch risers that can be attached to the four legs of the sofa to raise its height, making it easier to get in and out of. You can invest in couch assist rails to make it easier to stand up from the couch. Consider purchasing a caddy to keep commonly used items like the remote control and phone in. Re-arrange the furniture to allow easy access for wheelchairs or walkers. It is best to remove any area rugs in your living room as walkers can easily get caught up on it and potentially lead to a fall.

Laundry room:

Make sure that the space is not cluttered and there is enough space to move around. You can utilize a Reacher to help with moving clothes from the washer to the dryer. A top load washer is easier to use as it eliminates the need to bend over to remove the clothes once washed. A pedestal can be installed under your washer and dryer which will raise their height up reducing the chances of back strain. Instead of using heavy traditional liquid laundry detergent that can spill and can be difficult to pour, invest in detergent pods that can be easily tossed into the washer for cleaning. Keep all detergent and cleaners within reach. Invest in a rolling hamper to easily transport clothes from one room to another and conserve energy.

Chapter 15
My Memory is Getting Worse

Sara is at the grocery store and is in the checkout lane. The cashier smiles at her and asks if she found everything she was looking for. Sara replied, "You know, come to think of it, I had a hard time finding....," then she paused. She couldn't remember what she was going to say, she couldn't remember what she had a hard time finding. Her memory was not like it used to be. She looked up at the cashier and said, "Never mind, I found everything I needed."

There are various aspects of thinking and memory that may get affected with Parkinson's disease. Some major ones to highlight include:

- Paying attention or concentrating.

Have you been having problems participating in group conversations, or reading a book without getting distracted? Multitasking and problem-solving.

Do you get off balance if you are walking and talking at the same time? How about if your phone rings while you are balancing your checkbook?

I always recommend keeping a journal or memory book. It not only helps with the practice of writing bigger, but it also helps with jotting down activities as they happen — what was for breakfast, what happened after breakfast, etc. It builds up confidence as well because if someone asks what they did yesterday, they could always refer to their journal or memory book and have an answer. Using calendars, alarms and clocks is extremely helpful as well.

Reading sharpens your brain and keeps it active. Try doing crossword puzzles or playing games like Scrabble® and Taboo® that help exercise your brain to remember words. If you are having a tough time tracking the lines of a book, try using a ruler or a bookmark edge to guide each line. Try getting books that are large print.

In later stages of Parkinson's or for those who are older, Parkinson's Disease dementia is sometimes seen. People with PDD have trouble focusing and remembering things. Their judgment may be impaired. They may hallucinate and see people, objects or animals that are not there. The medications that help manage the symptoms of PDD are called cholinesterase inhibitors and can help with memory problems. Sleep medicines like melatonin® might also be prescribed by your doctor.

If a hallucination occurs, try switching the topic and see if that might assist with handling frustrations that occur because of a hallucination. Sometimes with PDD, there is difficulty with the day-night cycle. It is important not to correct a person with Parkinson's when a hallucination is occurring, it is best to go with the flow. Medication adjustments may not make the hallucinations disappear altogether, but it can make them less disturbing.

Establishing a set routine is important. At night, starting a "lights out" routine at the same hour every day, with all the curtains closed and lights turned off, can help a person understand that it is nighttime and time to sleep. On the contrary, during the day keep the curtains open and avoid naps and organize stimulating activities. Having calendars and clocks in each room can help to remember time of day. It always helps to talk out what you are doing and what is next. For example, let them know it is time to put on their shirt and pants and then it is time to go to church.

Door chimes or wireless door sensors can be used, and it will sound when the door is opened warning loved ones that a confused adult may be leaving the house. There are home alarm systems available that chime when a door is opened as well. Installing cameras inside and outside your home can also keep your loved one safe.

If you are noticing that you have been forgetful lately, it is good practice to say aloud what you are doing. For example, to help you remember that you have taken your medication, while you are doing it, say aloud, "I am taking my morning meds." When you go to your doctor's office, it is ok to write notes of what the doctor says so that you can remember all of it later.

Services like Lifeline® may be beneficial if you are concerned about your memory and safety. It is a twenty-four-hour emergency response system that can be hooked up to your phone. You will have either a wrist call button or a call button that can go around your neck which you always wear. If you need medical attention, all you need to do is push the button and the Response center will ask you the nature of your problem and will send help if needed.

A good night's sleep is particularly important, set a routine and sleeping schedule, even on weekends. This allows your brain and body time to reset and recharge. Try to avoid taking naps during the day and avoid drinks containing caffeine at least six hours before bedtime. A warm bath a few hours before bedtime raises your body temperature which helps with a good night's sleep. Meditation and relaxing breathing exercises can help you fall asleep as well. There are apps available now that can help you fall asleep by playing calming music or noises that can help you relax. White noise machines are effective for some people to help with sleep.

The loss of independence and abilities as well as changes in the brain chemistry can lead to feelings of depression. If you are having anxiety or are withdrawing from others, it is good to talk to your doctor. Some common antidepressants that can reduce depression include Effexor®, Prozac®, Lexapro® and Zoloft®. Attend a support group and talk to your friends, families, or trusted companion about how you are feeling. You are not alone in this process, you have people who care about you and are willing to help, all you need to do is ask.

Chapter 16

I Am Stooping, and My Posture is Getting Worse

Sara wakes up and is getting ready for the day. She looks at herself in the mirror and thinks to herself, 'Am I getting shorter?' She notices how slumped forward she is and feels her muscles are tighter. She remembers her high school days when she used to play basketball and how tall she was, what happened?

The spine or backbone is a flexible column that is made up of a series of bones stacked up one on top of the other called the vertebrae. This tall vertebral column is surrounded by muscles called the paraspinal muscles. The brain controls the tone of these muscles by sending an unconsciously generated message from the motor control area of the brain to the paraspinal muscles to maintain an upright posture. With Parkinson's this unconscious programming to the paraspinal muscles is affected, which causes the stooping. So, what can you do to overcome this? Yes, you are right! Consciously think about pulling your shoulders back and standing straight. Wall stands are a terrific way to improve your posture. Stand with your back against the wall and align your whole body (from head to feet) to it. Try to hold that posture for twenty seconds, relax and then repeat. This will train your mind to use this straight posture anytime you are standing or sitting up. Back squeeze is a good exercise to open up your chest and stretch your back. you can do a back squeeze anytime, anywhere. To do it, squeeze the shoulder blades back, as if you are trying to pinch a pen in place in the center of your back. Hold that squeeze for five seconds and repeat. You need to constantly think about standing straight for this to work—remember your unconscious circuit in your brain is not functioning properly—so use your conscious circuit and get yourself taller. Think big and straight with each stand and you will be surprised on how tall you really are!

Chapter 17

I Have a Referral for Physical Therapy, Occupational Therapy and Speech Therapy

Sara sits and waits for her name to be called at her doctor's office. She is embarrassed by her recent fall and is not looking forward to giving her doctor the details. The tremors start in her right hand and her breathing becomes more rapid. "Sara, we are ready for you," the nurse calls out. The doctor is very encouraging and ensures Sara that there is something she can do to help manage falls. He recommends that she start Physical Therapy, Occupational Therapy and Speech Therapy to help with some of her Parkinson's symptoms.

Exercise is a vital component for people with Parkinson's disease and it helps maintain balance and improve mobility. High-intensity exercises like boxing have shown to be beneficial as it drives brain change. The Parkinson's Outcomes Project® shows that people with Parkinson's disease who start exercising earlier in their disease course for a minimum of 2.5 hours per week, experience a slowed decline in quality of life than those who start later.

Remember, with Parkinson's, the neurons that produce the chemical neurotransmitter dopamine that helps with movement are damaged, and by the time Parkinson's symptoms appear there has already been an eighty percent depletion of these dopamine neurons. New connections need to be made and exercise has been shown effective in creating these new connections in the brain. Exercise regularly to help manage your symptoms of Parkinson's disease and change your brain. Your Physical Therapist, Occupational Therapist and Speech-language Pathologist will be able to prescribe individualized exercises that are right for you.

Physical therapists are experts in evaluating and treating musculoskeletal, neurological, and cardiovascular disorders. Physical therapists will perform a physical examination to gain a better understanding of your impairments and will establish goals with you to improve your independence. From there, they may use different techniques such as exercises, stretches, balance retraining, manual therapy and fall prevention strategies to help restore function and improve movement. They will prescribe you stretches to help with the slouched posture you may be having because of the tightness of your muscles around your shoulders and neck. Your physical therapist will help you walk better and will help you gain confidence in walking with bigger steps. Remember how we talked about that new neural pathway we are creating? Your Physical Therapist will remind you to keep using that pathway and do things bigger so that it becomes automatic.

With Parkinson's it is difficult to multitask so your therapist will challenge you to perform multiple things at the same time to help you improve in this area. For example, often patients have difficulty walking and talking at the same time. They get very distracted in crowded environments and are not able to focus on more than one thing. During sessions, I have the patients practice walking with bigger steps, usually I have markers on the ground so that they have a visual of how far each step needs to be. Then I add on to this by asking them to walk big while naming things along the way, encouraging them to look around for objects. I further add on by having them count by two's while walking big. My favorite is having them name all states that start with the letter M while continuing to walk big—their balance is really challenged with that one.

Your Physical therapist may also work on your stability and balance by having you walk around cones, over and on surfaces such as foam and other balance retraining strategies. Physical therapists will show you specialized exercises and stretches that will help with your Parkinson's symptoms. They also will help you improve your ability to transfer, climb steps and manage curbs and thresholds. As you can see, your Physical therapist will design a program that is individualized and geared towards managing your symptoms. There is an increasing recognition of the importance of performing more than one task simultaneously in daily life. This is called dual tasking and we do it all the time. Walking and talking, walking and carrying groceries, finding your way to an unfamiliar place while listening to your navigation give you directions and the list goes on and on. If you have Parkinson's, dual tasking is difficult as it requires a combination of motor and cognitive skills to perform these combined tasks. Your Physical therapist will be able to work on activities that are targeted both on motor function (like walking) and cognitive function (like counting by two's) simultaneously and help improve your ability to dual task.

Occupational therapists are experts who use therapeutic techniques to improve, a person's ability to perform everyday meaningful activities. Occupational Therapy helps you get back to the activities you normally perform from the time you wake up in the morning to the time you go to sleep. They help with gaining independence with tasks like getting out of bed, brushing your teeth, combing your hair, and getting dressed. Occupational therapists can assist patients in gaining independence with performing everyday tasks in a unique way using adaptive equipment as needed. They can assist with strengthening and stretching as well as making suggestions to modify the environment to get the job done more efficiently. Occupational therapists can suggest different tools and strategies to get patients independent with their activities of daily living.

Speech therapists or Speech-language Pathologists are experts who not only can help with speech and language disorders but can also assist with diagnosing and treating patients who need help with their thinking skills (cognition) and assist those with swallowing disorders. They can help with strategies to improve vocal quality for Parkinson's patients. People with Parkinson's may have trouble with getting food to their mouth, they may have leakage from their mouth, food getting stuck in the cheeks or may need extra time chewing. If you cough when eating or drinking, you may be at risk for aspiration pneumonia, which is the leading cause of death for people with Parkinson's disease. Your speech-language pathologist will teach you techniques for a safer swallow such as tucking in your chin. Sucking on ice fifteen minutes before your meal can help reduce any inflammation in your throat making swallowing easier. Your speech therapist may recommend that you get swallow tests called Modified Barium Swallow or maybe a FEES test to determine whether the food or liquid is entering a person's lungs, also known as aspiration. In this case, they may recommend a thickened liquid to prevent aspiration or a modified diet to assist with safe swallowing. They also can use electrical stimulation to re-train your swallowing muscles. Speech therapists can assist with teaching strategies to improve cognition, problem solving, processing and memory. The important thing is not to let speech difficulties prevent you from communicating with friends and loved ones. Masked face is common in people with Parkinson's—this means that there is a loss of facial expression, and it appears as if you have a mask on your face. Nonverbal gestures and expressions can lead to misunderstandings or miscommunication. If you are experiencing a masked face, make sure to exercise the muscles in your face— try smiling as big as you can, now hold that smile for five seconds. Next raise your eyebrows as high as you can and hold that position for five seconds. Try to stretch your jaw wide open and then hold. Finally try to flare your nostrils and hold for five seconds. All these exercises will build up those facial muscles and help improve your expression while talking with others. Another tip is to make a conscious effort to use your arms and hands to express yourself as you are talking with others, express verbally how you feel and what you are thinking.

Your neurologist may refer you to an excellent evidence-based therapy program for Parkinson's called Lee Silverman LSVT BIG® treatment. I use this treatment approach with my Parkinson's patients and have amazing results. After just one treatment session, I saw my patients performing better than when they came in. LSVT BIG® is a four-week program that includes four visits per week, a total of sixteen visits. The program focuses on high amplitude bigger movements that recalibrate your body to move normally with everyday activities and these exercises are specific to Parkinson's disease. Bigger the movement, the better. There are several evidence-based studies supporting the benefits of using this exercise approach. The voice component of LSVT is LSVT LOUD® which focuses on recalibrating the brain to speak louder. Parkinson's Wellness Recovery® (PWR) is another evidence-based treatment program for Parkinson's that consists of a set of movements that your PT or OT perform with you to help better manage the physical and neurological effects of Parkinson's disease. When you seek out treatment for Parkinson's, my recommendation is to ask for an LSVT BIG® or PWR® therapist for PT and OT and to ask for a LSVT LOUD® speech-language pathologist.

Chapter 18

My Therapist Recommended I Join a Gym and Do Aerobic Exercise

Sara joined her community YWCA® at the advice of her Physical Therapist. She looked around and saw all the exercise equipment she could take advantage of. She was excited to start this new regimen and improve her physical and mental well-being. She was already noticing huge improvements with her therapy sessions, and now she could take this one step further by incorporating exercise into her daily routine.

There is substantial evidence that shows that aerobic exercises help to prevent age-related loss of muscle, bone, and brain volume—keeping the body and mind healthy. Exercise has also been shown to be good for treating depression. Aerobic exercise is a physical exercise that increases your pulse, makes you sweat and makes you tired. Exercises need to be challenging to get that brain re-wired and for that new neural pathway to light up. Before starting with aerobic exercise, talk to your neurologist about optimization of carbidopa/levodopa dosage. Exercise goes best when you are in your levodopa on-state. It is harder to exercise when your levodopa is starting to wear off.

What are some aerobic exercises? Walking is one of the best activities out there, ideally at a brisk pace. Try walking on a treadmill every day or set a routine to walk around the neighborhood every evening. Treadmill walking has been shown to be beneficial for improving both gait speed and aerobic fitness. Other activities such as gardening, cycling, boxing, and dancing can make you sweaty and are good options for aerobic activities.

Utilize the exercise equipment in your gym. Instead of adding more weights, do more repetitions. If you have a pool, swimming is also an excellent form of aerobic exercise. I have found recumbent bikes and Nu-step® bikes very beneficial in improving coordination, postural stability, and generalized muscle strength. Any activity that gets you sweaty and makes your heart rate rise is aerobic exercise. Choose activities that are right for you and that you will continue doing. Have a few backups so that in case you get bored with one aerobic activity, you can switch up and do another. Get registered with a boxing fitness class, boxing has been shown to improve performance in people with Parkinson's. Do not hold your breath

Chapter 18: My Therapist Recommended I Join a Gym and Do Aerobic Exercise

when you exercise, incorporate deep breathing into your exercise regimen. Inhale and exhale as you perform your aerobic exercises, check your heart rate, and take rest breaks as needed. It is easy to talk yourself out of exercises, and to produce excuses. Push yourself harder and harder and set goals. When you start seeing the results, you will be determined to continue.

Chapter 19
Reclaim Your Life and Don't Give Up

※

When Sara was at her doctor's office, they were able to provide her with a pamphlet of Parkinson's support services in the area. Sara was surprised to see all the free classes, groups and social and enrichment support programs that were available to her. She knew it would be good to share her experiences with people who were going through the same thing. Sara decides to attend a support class that provided an opportunity to swap stories and share resources which was therapeutic to her; it helped her realize that she was not alone in this process. My patients are shocked as well when I provide them with information on all the perks of the Houston Area Parkinson's Society® in our area. They have group exercise classes, boxing classes, speech classes, support groups and other resources free of charge to people living with

Parkinson's. There are support services available to every state. If you go to Parkinson.org® and type in your zip code, you will be able to view all resources available in your area. You can also visit the American Parkinson's Disease Association® website for more information on Parkinson's. Caretakers and family members also benefit from sharing questions and concerns with others going through the same process. Look up the support services in your area, get registered and take advantage of all they have to offer. There are also online support groups such as The Parkinson's Buddy Network®, Neurotalk®, PatientsLikeMe, etc. that have a Parkinson's forum.

The entire process of Parkinson's may be difficult—from the onset of symptoms to the official diagnosis to seeking out treatment. You may be overwhelmed with emotions and feelings of despair, anger, grief, denial, and hope. Talk to your doctor of you are having a tough time regulating your emotions. Don't isolate yourself, remember you have a support system waiting for you and rooting for you. The resources are available, all you need to do is embrace them!

Chapter 20
You've Got This!

It's Thanksgiving again and it has been over a year since Sara received the news that she had Parkinson's. Her family has come to stay for the weekend. Sara looks around and reflects upon all the hurdles she had to overcome this past year. She remembers the day that she walked into the neurologist's office and heard the words, "Try this medication, you may have Parkinson's." So much has happened over the past year. Sara thinks back to the days she was up and down, mostly down and she knew she had to find a community of support to feel less alone, so she joined a few community support groups to get involved with the Parkinson's community. That provided so much relief, for the first time she could relate to people who understood exactly what she was going through. Sara started physical therapy, occupational therapy and speech therapy and was surprised how much better she could move and speak. Sara has finally embraced her diagnosis; she knows that she will continue to have good and not-so-good days. But this whole journey of life is uncertain, throwing curves all the time with or without Parkinson's. Sara looks over at her children in the kitchen, busy preparing the dinner feast; she raised them well and is proud of each one of their accomplishments. She glances at her precious grandchildren who are her pride and joy, playing video games in the living room. She recognizes how blessed she is with a family who loves and supports her. She finally understands that this disease does not have control over her, she has control over it! She is determined to be active and to be positive, taking each day as it comes.

You need to keep being who you are, don't compare yourself to others—just do what you can do and embrace your diagnosis. You have the power to help manage your symptoms, your mind is a powerful thing. Do what you can when you can and be proud that you are not giving up. Life with Parkinson's is possible. The only proven thing that slows the progression of the disease is exercise, so instead of being discouraged, get out there and just do it! It may be hard at first but be consistent and you will get results. Make exercise a part of your life, set an alarm for when it is time to do your exercises daily. Treat exercises the same way you treat your medications—you need your medicines to help your body, you need the exercises to reduce your symptoms. There is going to be good days and bad days, begin each day with a positive outlook and the confidence that you have power over your mind. It's not how many times you get knocked down, it's how many times you gained the strength to stand back up. Sometimes you must stop worrying, wondering, and doubting. Trust the process, gain confidence in your abilities, there is nothing too difficult to achieve if you set your mind to it. Believing opens the doors to possibilities—life is what you make of it, never take it for granted. Reclaim your life, you've got this!

Resources

Apps

Speak Up App for Parkinson's
1930 6th Avenue South, Suite 303
Seattle, WA, 98134
206-325-5383
www.sandcastle-web.com/

Loud and Clear App
https://loudandclear.io/

Beats Medical Parkinson's Therapy App
www.beatsmedical.com/parkinsons

Resources for Adaptive equipment and Assistive Devices

U-Step Walker
8048 Monticello Ave.
Skokie, IL 60076
1-800-558-7837
www.ustep.com

Elastic Shoelaces
Lock laces
www.locklaces.com

Gyenno Parkinson Spoon
www.gyenno.com

Weighted Utensils, Dressing Adaptive equipment, Abdominal binder
Performance Health
28100 Torch Parkway, Suite 700
Warrenville, IL 60555
630-393-6000
https://performancehealth.com

Compression Stockings
Jobst USA
www.jobst-usa.com

Luxe Bidet®
www.luxebidet.com
858-360-7780

Bottom Buddy®
945 Reservoir Road
Madison Township, PA 18444
hygieneease@gmail.com

Rocker knife
Allegro Medical
360 Veterans Parkway, Suite 115
Bolingbrook, IL 60440-4607
United States
1-800-861-3211

www.allegromedical.com/

Leg lifters, Weighted hand gloves, Couch handrails, Couch risers
The Wright Stuff Inc.
111 Harris Street
Crystal Springs, MS 39059
601-892-3115
www.mobility-aids.com

Dycem
Dycem Corporation
1725 Hughes Landing Blvd, Suite 865,
The Woodlands, Texas 77380
contact@dycem.com

Plate Guard
AliMed, Inc.
297 High Street
Dedham, MA 02026
800-225-2610
Weighted wide grip pens, Universal Cuff Adaptive Utensil Holder, Bed Rails
Rehab Mart, LLC
1353 Athens Hwy
Elbertson, GA 30677
800-827-8283

Walker Tray
Medline Industries
800-633-5463

Car handle assist
Vive Health
800-487-3808

Speech Amplifiers
Chattervox
847-816-8580
www.chattervox.com

Walker glide skis
Nova Medical Walker Skis
PO Box 80729
RSM, CA-92688
949-713-1400
www.senior.com

Evidence based Exercise Programs for Parkinson's

LSVT Global
4720 N. Oracle St., Ste 100
Tucson, AZ 85705
888-438-5788.
www.lsvtglobal.com

Parkinson's Wellness Recovery
4343 N. Oracle Rd #173
Tucson, AZ 85705

520-591-5346
www.pwr4life.org

Home Adaptation Resources

Consumer's Guide to Home Adaptation
Adaptive Environments
374 Congress Street, Suite 301
Boston, MA 02210
617-695-1225
www.adaptiveenvironments.org

Home Comfort Solutions, LLC
13121 Louetta Road #500
Cypress, TX 77429
713-623-1388
www.elderoptionsoftexas.com

Meal Delivery Services

Meals on Wheels
National Office
1414 Prince Street, Suite 302
Alexandria, VA 22314
703-548-5558
www.mowaa.org

Other Resources

Duopa
1-844-438-6720
www.duopa.com

Lifeline
800-380-3111
www.lifelinesys.com

Talking Pill Bottle
Easy Street Co.
509 Birchwood Court
Raymore, MO 64083
800-959-3279
www.easystreetco.com

The Breather
Northern Speech Services
325 Meecher Rd.
PO Box 1247
Gaylord, MI-49735
888-337-3866
www.northernspeech.com

Resources to learn more about Parkinson's

American Parkinson Disease Association
PO Box 61420
Staten Island, NY 10306

800-223-2732
www.apdaparkinson.org

The Michael J. Fox Foundation for Parkinson's Research
Grand Central Station
P.O. Box 4777
New York, NY 10163
800-708-7644
www.michaeljfox.org

National Institute of Disability and Rehabilitation Research
ABLEDATA
U.S. Department of Education
8630 Fenton Street, MD 20910
800-227-0216
www.abledata.com

National Parkinson Foundation, Inc.
Bob Hope Parkinson Research Center
Bop Hope Road
1501 NW 9th Avenue
Miami, FL 33136-1494
800-327-4545
www.parkinson.org

Parkinson Disease Foundation, Inc.
1359 Broadway, Suite 1509
New York, NY 10018
800-457-6676

www.pdf.org

Parkinson's Outcome Project
Parkinson's Foundation
200 SE 1st Street, Ste 800
Miami, FL 33131
800-473-4636
www.parkinson.org/advancing-research/our-research/parkinsons-outcomes-project

Support Groups

Houston Area Parkinson's Society
2700 Southwest Fwy #296
Houston, TX 77098
713-626-7114
www.hapsonline.org

Parkinson's Buddy Network
www.parkinsonsbuddynetwork.michaeljfox.org

NeuroTalk
www.neurotalk.org

PatientsLikeMe

www.patientslikeme.com

References

About PWR! – Parkinson wellness recovery. (n.d.). PWR! Retrieved October 17, 2022, from https://www.pwr4life.org/about/

Admin, A. (2018, April 6). ADA Solutions. ADA Solutions, LLC. https://adatile.com/all-you-need-to-know-about-ada-curb-ramp-requirements/

American Parkinson Disease Association: Hope in progress. (2017, January 15). American Parkinson Disease Association. https://www.apdaparkinson.org/

Bryans, L. A., Palmer, A. D., Anderson, S., Schindler, J., & Graville, D. J. (2021). The impact of Lee Silverman Voice Treatment (LSVT LOUD®) on voice, communication, and participation: Findings from a prospective, longitudinal study. Journal of Communication Disorders, 89, 106031. https://doi.org/10.1016/j.jcomdis.2020.106031

Custom Native iOS App Developed for Seattle NWPF. (n.d.). Seattle, WA. Retrieved October 17, 2022, from https://www.sandcastle-web.com/services/mobile-solutions/iosandroid-apps/speak-up-for-parkinsons-ios-app/

Deep brain stimulation. (2021, August 8). Johns Hopkins Medicine. https://www.hopkinsmedicine.org/health/treatment-tests-and-therapies/deep-brain-stimulation

Drugs & medications. (n.d.). WebMD. Retrieved October 17, 2022, from https://www.webmd.com/drugs/2/drug-3394-41/carbidopa-levodopa-oral/carbidopa-levodopa-oral/details

Fayyaz, M., Jaffery, S. S., Anwer, F., Zil-E-Ali, A., & Anjum, I. (2018). The effect of physical activity in Parkinson's disease: A mini review. Cureus, 10(7). https://doi.org/10.7759/cureus.2995

GYENNO SPOON. (n.d.). Retrieved October 17, 2022, from https://www.gyenno.com/spoon-en

Hallucinations/Delusions. (n.d.). Parkinson's Foundation. Retrieved October 17, 2022, from https://www.parkinson.org/understanding-parkinsons/symptoms/non-movement-symptoms/hallucinations-delusions

In-Step mobility, creator of the u-step walker for Parkinson's disease. (2017, July 6). Ustep. https://www.ustep.com/

Isaacson, S., O'Brien, A., Lazaro, J. D., Ray, A., & Fluet, G. (2018). The JFK BIG study: The impact of LSVT BIG® on dual task walking
and mobility in persons with Parkinson's disease. Journal of

Physical Therapy Science, 30(4).

https://doi.org/10.1589/jpts.30.636

Jobst USA. (n.d.). Jobst. Retrieved October 17, 2022, from

https://www.jobst-usa.com/

Körner Gustafsson, J., Södersten, M., Ternström, S., & Schalling, E. (2018). Long-term effects of Lee Silverman Voice Treatment on daily voice use in Parkinson's disease as measured with a portable voice accumulator. Logopedics Phoniatrics Vocology, 44(3), 124–133. https://doi.org/10.1080/14015439.2018.1435718

Laces®, L. (n.d.). The original elastic no-tie shoelaces. Lock Laces®. Retrieved October 17, 2022, from https://www.locklaces.com/

Li, Y., Tan, M., Fan, H., Wang, E. Q., Chen, L., Li, J., Chen, X., & Liu, H. (2021). Neurobehavioral effects of LSVT® LOUD on auditory-vocal integration in Parkinson's disease: A preliminary study. Frontiers in Neuroscience, 0.

https://doi.org/10.3389/fnins.2021.624801

Loud and Clear – Voice fitness for people with Parkinson's. (n.d.). Retrieved October 17, 2022, from https://loudandclear.io/

Ltd, B. M. (2014, April 26). Beats medical Parkinson's app. App Store. https://apps.apple.com/us/app/beats-medical-parkinsons-app/id866567480

LUXE bidet — premium quality bidets. (n.d.). LUXE Bidet.

    Retrieved October 17, 2022, from https://luxebidet.com/

Meals on Wheels. (2019, August 17). Homage.

    https://homage.org/nutrition/meals-on-wheels/

Micrographia. (2017, March 1). ParkinsonsDisease.Net.

    https://parkinsonsdisease.net/symptoms/micrographia-handwriting

National Institute on Disability and Rehabilitation Research, Office of Special Education and Rehabilitative Services (OSERS). (n.d.). NIDCD. Retrieved October 17, 2022, from https://www.nidcd.nih.gov/directory/national-institute-disability-and-rehabilitation-research-office-special-education-and

NeuroTalk forums - Neurological support groups. (n.d.). NeuroTalk.

    Retrieved October 17, 2022, from https://www.neurotalk.org/

"Off" time in Parkinson's disease. (n.d.). The Michael J. Fox Foundation for Parkinson's Research | Parkinson's Disease. Retrieved October 17, 2022, from https://www.michaeljfox.org/time-parkinsons-disease

O'Sullivan, S. B., Schmitz, T. J., & Fulk, G. D. (2013). Physical rehabilitation. F A Davis Company.

Parkinsonfoundation.org -. (n.d.). Parkinsonfoundation.Org. Retrieved October 17, 2022, from https://parkinsonfoundation.org/

Parkinson's 101. (n.d.). The Michael J. Fox Foundation for Parkinson's Research | Parkinson's Disease. Retrieved October 17, 2022, from https://www.michaeljfox.org/parkinsons-101

Parkinson's disease & DUOPATM (carbidopa/levodopa). (n.d.). Official Patient Site. Retrieved October 17, 2022, from https://www.duopa.com/

Parkinson's disease - Symptoms and causes. (2022, July 8). Mayo Clinic. https://www.mayoclinic.org/diseases-conditions/parkinsons-disease/symptoms-causes/syc-20376055

Parkinson's outcomes project. (n.d.). Parkinson's Foundation. Retrieved October 17, 2022, from https://www.parkinson.org/advancing-research/our-research/parkinsons-outcomes-project

PatientsLikeMe. (n.d.). PatientsLikeMe. Retrieved October 17, 2022, from https://www.patientslikeme.com/

PeopleGrove. (n.d.). Retrieved October 17, 2022, from https://parkinsonsbuddynetwork.michaeljfox.org/v2/

Peterka, Odorfer, Schwab, Volkmann, & Zeller. (2020). LSVT-BIG therapy in Parkinson's disease: Physiological evidence for proprioceptive recalibration. BMC Neurology, 20(1), 1–8. https://doi.org/10.1186/s12883-020-01858-2

Physical therapy for Parkinson's. (n.d.). LSVT BIG. Retrieved October 17, 2022, from https://www.lsvtglobal.com/LSVTBig

radair@mediaateam.com. (2022, March 18). Home - Houston Area Parkinson Society. My WordPress. https://hapsonline.org/

Schwarz, S. P. (2006). Parkinson's disease: 300 tips for making life easier, 2nd edition. Demos Medical Publishing.

Speech therapy for Parkinson's disease and other conditions. (n.d.). LSVT Global. Retrieved October 17, 2022, from https://www.lsvtglobal.com/LSVTLoud

Talking prescription bottles can make life easier. (n.d.). CVS Health. Retrieved October 17, 2022, from https://www.cvshealth.com/news-and-insights/articles/talking-prescription-bottles-can-make-life-easier

The Breather®. (n.d.). Respiratory Muscle Training Device. Retrieved October 17, 2022, from https://www.northernspeech.com/rmt-respiratory-muscle-training/the-breather/

Tsukita, K., Sakamaki-Tsukita, H., & Takahashi, R. (2022). Long-term effect of regular physical activity and exercise habits in patients with early parkinson disease. Neurology, 98(8), e859–e871. https://doi.org/10.1212/WNL.0000000000013218

About the Author:

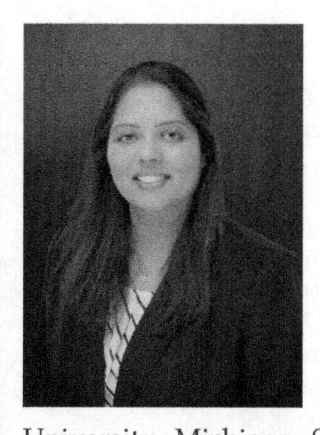

Susha Thomas PT, DPT, C/NDT is a Physical Therapist who has specializations in Parkinson's and Stroke rehabilitation. She has been treating Parkinson's patients since 2002 and received her Doctor of Physical Therapy degree from Wayne State University, Michigan. She is an active volunteer with the Houston Area Parkinson's Society. She serves as the Director of Therapy Operations and Program Chair for Parkinson's at an Inpatient Rehabilitation Hospital. She mentors and helps bring awareness to the disease, dispelling stigma while advocating for the PD community. She resides with her husband and children in Houston, Texas. This book has a personalized touch and includes illustrations drawn by her children Jaden and Elena.

INDEX

a long-handled dustpan, 77
Abdominal binders, 58
activities of daily living, 52, 62
adaptive equipment, 2, 36, 47, 55, 91
adaptive tools, 54
aerobic exercises, 94, 95
aerobic fitness, 95
alarm, 9, 16, 101
alarms, 18, 81
amantadine, 12
Amazon echo, 74
American Parkinson's Disease Association®, 98
anger, 51, 98
antidepressants, 68, 84
anxiety, 84
apps, 26, 45, 84
aspiration, 91
aspiration pneumonia, 91
assistive devices, 63
backbone, 85
balance, 7, 10, 17, 50, 59, 66, 68, 73, 81, 87, 88
Balance, 66, 68
bathroom, 51, 72, 73, 74, 75
Beats Medical Parkinson's app, 45
bed rails, 78
bedroom, 76, 78
bidet, 75
blood pressure, 13, 56, 57, 58, 59, 60, 68
blood pressure cuff, 57
boxing, 87, 95, 97

brain, 3, 4, 5, 11, 12, 16, 19, 20, 21, 22, 23, 25, 27, 31, 36, 39, 40, 43, 44, 45, 53, 58, 62, 65, 81, 83, 84, 85, 87, 88, 93, 94
  basal ganglia, 3
  substantia nigra, 3
brain circuit, 44
button, 17, 51, 67, 77, 83
button hook, 51
caffeine, 83
calendars, 81, 82
cane, 46
car, 15, 20, 38, 47, 73
car handle assist, 73
Carbidopa/Levodopa, 12
Carbidopa-levodopa, 16
cardiac output, 58
caregiver, 26, 37, 53
cholinesterase inhibitors, 82
clocks, 81, 82
cognition, 91
compression stockings, 57
confusion, 17, 56
conscious circuit, 86
constipation, 11, 13
coordination, 7, 11
couch assist rails, 79
couch risers, 79
couch risers., 67
cues, 53
curbs, 90
dance, 68
Deep Brain Stimulation, 12
Dehydration, 13, 59

117

denial, 98
depressed, 10
depression., 84, 94
depth perception, 46
despair, 98
disabilities, 47
doorknobs, 74
doorway, 46, 76
Doorways, 76
dopamine, 4, 5, 6, 7, 12, 16, 19, 25, 30, 62, 88
dopamine agonists, 12
dressing, 50, 54, 62
dressing sticks, 54
drooling, 11, 65
droxidopa, 59
dual tasking, 90
Duopa, 13, 16, 107
Dycem, 64, 105
dyskinesia, 12
dystonia, 12
eating, 13, 62, 64, 65, 91
Effexor®, 84
elastic shoelaces, 52
elastic thread, 51
elastic waistbands, 50
electrical stimulation, 92
emotions, 13, 98
endurance, 68
energy conservation, 75
exercise, 1, 42, 68, 81, 86, 88, 92, 94, 95, 97, 101
Fall recovery, 69
falls, 7, 68, 72, 74, 87
fearful of falling, 66
FEES test, 92
festinating gait, 43
flexibility, 68
fludrocortisone, 60
freezing, 1, 12, 44, 45, 46, 53
gait speed, 95
General home safety, 72
Google mini, 74
grab bars, 75
grief, 98

grip, 33, 52, 62, 64, 74, 105
GYENNO Parkinson spoon and fork, 63
hallucination, 82
handheld shower, 75
handrails, 67, 77, 104
handwriting, 1, 7, 9, 10, 19, 30, 31, 32, 33
High-intensity exercises, 87
home improvements, 72
home monitoring devices, 67
hope, 25, 98
Houston Area Parkinson's Society®, 97
incontinence, 78
incontinence briefs, 78
intense, 36, 50, 52
involuntary, 12
involuntary movements, 7, 12
journal, 18, 81
kitchen, 66, 77, 101
larynx, 25
laser light, 47
Leg lifters, 36, 104
Lexapro®, 84
Lifeline®, 83
lighting, 74
living room, 24, 78, 101
long shoehorns, 54
Loud and Clear App, 26, 103
low blood pressure, 56
LSVT BIG®, 93
LSVT LOUD®, 93
lungs, 27, 92
markers, 31, 43
masked face, 10, 92
Masked face, 92
meditation, 68
melatonin®, 82
memory, 80, 81, 82, 83, 92
metronomes, 45
micrographia, 30, 32
Midodrine, 59
Modified Barium Swallow, 92
Motion detector light switches, 74

motor control area of the brain, 85
movement, 3, 5, 6, 12, 16, 19, 31, 35, 36, 38, 39, 40, 44, 45, 50, 51, 52, 62, 88
multitask, 39, 89
Multitasking, 81
muscle strength, 11
music, 45, 53, 84
Nest®, 74
neural pathway, 20, 21, 23, 25, 31, 89
neurologist, 11, 12, 13, 15, 42, 93, 95, 100
neurons, 88
neuroplasticity, 20, 36
Neurotalk®, 98
neurotransmitter, 3, 88
neurotransmitter), 3
occupational therapist, 33, 88
on time, 15, 17, 18, 50
orthostatic hypotension, 57, 59
pants, 51, 82
paraspinal muscles, 85
Parkinson.org®, 98
Parkinson's Disease dementia, 81
Parkinson's Wellness Recovery® (PWR), 93
PatientsLikeMe, 98, 110
peak performance, 17
Peer support, 69
Pen grips, 33
perception, 46
physical therapist, 24, 88, 89
Physical Therapist, 1, 94, 118
pill boxes, 17
pill-rolling tremor, 62
pill-rolling tremors, 7
Plate guards, 63
pocketing of food, 65
poor balance, 6
posture, 7, 85, 89
pressure injury, 47
problem solving, 92
problem-solving, 81
processing, 13, 92
progressive disorder, 1

Prozac®, 84
pyridostigmine, 60
quality of life, 1, 12, 14, 88
raised toilet seat, 75
ramp, 77
reachers, 54
Re-arrange furniture, 72
recovery position, 58
reflexes, 11
resources, 97, 99
retrain, 20
Retrain, 46
rigidity, 6, 7, 17
rocker knife, 63
rocker-panel switches, 74
roll, 36, 37
routine, 68, 82, 83, 94
Rytary, 16
Seatbelt extenders, 73
self-care activities, 53
sensation, 11
shaking, 10, 51, 63
shirt, 10, 49, 50, 53, 82
shoelaces, 52
shower chair, 75
Shuffle, 42
shuffling, 11, 12
Sinemet, 16
sleep, 62, 68, 82, 83
small steps., 11
smaller movements, 6, 7, 19
smart home speakers, 74
smell, 10
sock aides, 54
socks, 52
Speak Up for Parkinson's, 26
speech amplifiers, 28
speech-language pathologist, 26, 88, 91, 93
spinal cord, 11
stability, 47, 73, 89
stairlift, 76
stairs, 46, 73, 76
Steps to get off of the floor, 69
stiff, 7, 9, 35, 46

strength, 68, 102
stretching, 50, 51, 68, 91
Stretching, 35
stuck, 10, 21, 35, 38, 40, 44, 45, 49, 91
support group, 84
swallowing, 11, 16, 65, 91
symptoms, 1, 6, 7, 10, 11, 12, 13, 15, 16, 17, 56, 57, 59, 82, 87, 88, 90, 98, 101
Tai chi, 68
Talking pill bottles®, 17
target, 6, 19, 20, 26, 43, 45
The Breather, 27, 108
The Parkinson's Buddy Network®, 98
The Parkinson's Outcomes Project®, 88
thickened liquid, 92
threshold, 46
thresholds, 45, 90
throw rugs, 72
toilet safety frame, 75
tremors, 6, 7, 16, 17, 33, 51, 52, 61, 62, 63, 64, 87
tub transfer bench, 75

unconscious circuit, 86
Universal cuff utensil holders, 64
U-step walker, 47
Velcro, 50, 52, 54
vertebrae, 85
Visual biofeedback, 51
visual feedback, 26, 33, 53
vitamin D, 13
vocal cords, 25, 27, 28
voice, 1, 7, 10, 19, 24, 25, 26, 27, 28, 45, 93
Walker slides, 68
Walker trays, 68
walkers, 68, 73, 79
walking, 1, 7, 15, 16, 42, 43, 44, 45, 47, 66, 69, 81, 89, 95
wearing-off, 17
Weighted cups and plates, 64
Weighted pens, 33, 64
Weighted utensils, 63, 64
Weighted wide grip pens, 64, 105
wheelchair, 47, 76
yoga, 68
zipper pulls, 54
Zoloft®, 84

Made in the USA
Coppell, TX
07 August 2024